DATE DUE

MY 4 '98			
NO 4 '99			
AP 22 '02			
AG 4 '03			
BR 21 06			
MY 27 '09			

DEMCO 38-296

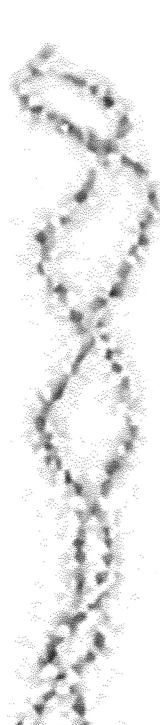

Does It Run in the Family?

A Consumer's Guide to DNA Testing for Genetic Disorders

Doris Teichler Zallen

Rutgers University Press

New Brunswick, New Jersey, and London

Library of Congress Cataloging-in-Publication data

Zallen, Doris Teichler.
  Does it run in the family? : a consumer's guide to DNA testing for
genetic disorders / Doris Teichler Zallen.
    p.   cm.
  Includes bibliographical references and index.
  ISBN 0-8135-2446-6 (cloth : alk. paper)
  1. Genetic disorders—Diagnosis—Popular works.   I. Title.
RB155.6.T45   1997
616'.042—dc21   96-49677
                                                            CIP

British Cataloging-in-Publication information available

Manufactured in the United States of America

For my family
Richard, Jennifer, and Avram
and
for all the families
who so generously shared their experiences

Contents

Preface and Acknowledgments

E ach new era in medicine has brought with it both promise and problems. At the start, hopes arise that we can, at last, defeat disease and improve the quality of human life. Invariably, this is followed by the realization that the new medical advances have themselves created new difficulties and new dilemmas. So it is with the era of genetic medicine on which we have just embarked.

We are now in a period of rapidly deepening knowledge of human genetics. This knowledge permits an unprecedented understanding of the relationship between our genes and our health. It offers the promise of better treatments for genetic disorders, perhaps (someday) even cures. It gives us the genetic test, a new way of gaining information about ourselves. But genetic information often includes an element of uncertainty. And genetic information is laden with baggage. This baggage is historical, ethical, emotional, social. In some circumstances, the information can be useful and important; in some, it can be trifling or insignificant. And in some circumstances, it can be harmful.

My own introduction to the complex tangle of issues surrounding genetic tests came very personally. In the early 1980s, while a researcher at the University of Rochester School of Medicine, I was working on developing some early forms of genetic linkage testing. In my contact with the families taking part in those studies, I became keenly aware of the mixed effects that this new form of genetic testing could have, even for different members of the same family. Since 1983, as a faculty member in an interdisciplinary humanities and science-studies program at Virginia Tech, I have concentrated on examining the ethical, historical, and public policy aspects of genetics.

This book is the result of an ongoing effort to understand the development and potential of new genetic tests, to determine how genetic information is made available, and to learn how decisions about the use of tests are made. The emphasis here is on the newest type of genetic testing, the so-called DNA tests that are capable of examining the genetic material itself. These tests are rapidly coming into wide use as a result of intense research efforts under way throughout the world. Although I focus on the DNA tests, much of what I describe here also applies to the more traditional forms of genetic testing which preceded DNA testing.

The book is written for a general audience. As genetic tests find their way into medical practice, many of us will increasingly be faced with making choices about whether or not we want to use them. This book is intended to provide some insight into how genetic testing decisions are made, as well as some information about what resources are available to assist people in making these decisions.

I am greatly indebted to all the people who participated in the interviews that provided the material on which much of this book is based. Julie Gordon of MUMS (Mothers United for Moral Support), Abbey Meyers of NORD (National Organization for Rare Disorders), and Janet Glover-Kerkvliet (Foundation Fighting Blindness) provided assistance that enabled me to contact individuals and families throughout the country. National and regional Breast Cancer Action groups placed notices in their newsletters for me. Thanks to the help of these organizations and groups, I was able to speak to individuals in a wide variety of genetic situations and to learn how people do and do not obtain genetic information. Counselors associated with genetic service units at several medical centers also helped arrange interviews with their clients. This allowed me to learn how decisions are made once genetic information is received. The eighty interviews which resulted provided the opportunity to gain vital firsthand accounts of a wide spectrum of genetic issues. All of those interviewed were extraordinarily willing to share their histories, their experiences, and their evaluations of genetic matters. They were generous beyond measure in making time available in their own very active lives. I have tried to represent, honestly and authentically, what they conveyed in those interviews. I have altered details (but not substance) only in order to protect their privacy.

Interviews with genetic professionals provided many key insights that could only have come from those working on the front lines. I particularly wish to thank: Robin L. Bennett, Judith Benkendorf, Linda M. Brzustowicz, Robert J. Desnick, Helen Donis-Keller, Robert Erickson, Gerald Feldman, Jeanette Felix, Merry Ferre, Daniel Finkelstein, Vicky L. Funanage, Judy Garza, Janet Glover-Kerkvliet, Ann Jewell, Matthew Lubin, Maria J. Mascari, Karen Miller, Kathleen Monroe, Arno G. Motulsky, Robert Murray, Jane Peterson, Pam Plumeau, Barbara Quinton, Leslie J. Raffel, Vincent M. Riccardi, Jennifer Robinson, Gladys Rosenthal, Pat Schnatterly, and Stephen Warren. Conversations with Robert C. Baumiller, Colleen D. Clements, Donald Lindberg, Philip Noguchi, Edward L. Schacht, and William Shannon have permitted me to consider a fuller range of issues related to genetic testing.

A symposium I organized for the 1988 American Association for the Advancement of Science (AAAS) annual meeting in Boston, on "Human Linkage Testing: The New Ethical Issues," provided one of the first opportunities to examine the then emerging forms of DNA testing with the views of a public audience. This symposium was cosponsored by the AAAS Committee on Scientific Freedom and Responsibility and by the American Society of Human Genetics. Many of the aspects of DNA testing examined by the audience and the symposium presenters (Haig H. Kazazian, Jr., Eric S. Lander, Mark Lappé, J. Robert Nelson, and Philip R. Reilly) appear in this book.

My membership on the Recombinant DNA Advisory Committee (the "RAC") of the National Institutes of Health from 1992–1995 and, before that, on the Human Gene Therapy Subcommittee of the RAC enabled me to see firsthand the progress being made in developing new types of treatments for genetic disorders.

Research trips to the U.K. in 1991, and to Canada in 1994, provided the opportunity to gain a cross-national perspective. I especially appreciate the in-depth discussions I had with Michael Baraitser, Christine

Barnes, Frances Beards, Caroline Berry, (Sir) Walter Bodmer, Sue Cox, Shirley Dalby, Kay E. Davies, Peter Harris, the late Anita E. Harding, Michael Hayden, Shirley Hodgson, Alison Lashwood, William McKellin, Helen Middleton-Price, Anthony P. Monaco, Victoria Murday, Marcus Pembrey, Sarah Ross, Mary J. Seller, Gwen Turner, Margaret Van-Altaan, Andrew O. M. Wilkie, and Robert Williamson.

Support received from the National Endowment for the Humanities (FT-37821-93) and a research leave provided by Virginia Tech made the analysis and writing possible. A travel grant awarded by the College of Arts and Sciences at Virginia Tech defrayed the cost of research and interview trips.

Richard Doherty, Marjorie Grene, Jennifer Zallen, and Richard Zallen valiantly read and offered detailed comments on the entire manuscript. Wendy Farkas, Julie Gordon, Joy Harvey, Carol McManus, Vincent Riccardi, Maurie Temple, Barry and Felicia Volkman, and Avi Zallen offered comments on selected portions. Students in the "Humanities and the Life Sciences" course at Virginia Tech provided their reactions to Chapters Four and Five. Michael Volkman, an independent disability-rights consultant and advocate, helped with the material on the Americans with Disabilities Act in Chapter Six. Louise Elbaum of the Great Lakes Regional Genetics Group supplied consent forms that were helpful for Chapter Seven. Rebecca Scheckler provided suggestions for the Appendix and Chris Hays Dove gave careful feedback on the Glossary. The figures in this book have benefited from the excellent art work of June Mullins. Karen Reeds at Rutgers University Press has been an outstanding editor, bringing this project along from its inception. I am grateful to all these people for their criticism and advice. Much as I have relied on their knowledge, wisdom, and experience, I have nonetheless stubbornly resisted some of their recommendations.

This book has only been possible because of the boundless kindness, continuous encouragement, incredible constancy, and, more often than I care to admit, the personal sacrifice of my own family. To my husband, Richard, my children, Jennifer and Avi, and my mother, Bessie Teichler, go my love and a gratitude that words are inadequate to express.

A Word on Words

Throughout this book, I have used the word "consumer" to refer to individuals who are candidates for genetic testing, who need information about genetic disorders, or who are interested in finding out whether genetic testing could be useful to them at some point in their lives. I realize that the word "consumer" is inadequate. It conveys no sense of the anguish and stress experienced by many of those who are forced to confront a genetic disorder. Still, in the absence of any adequate term, I have found that "consumer" is preferred by many lay people and genetic professionals alike.

I have also chosen to use the word "normal" as a shorthand for the standard, most common, form of a gene, chromosome, or protein. This usage, while convenient, obscures the fact that much variation occurs in nature. There are many nonstandard, uncommon forms of genes, chromosomes, and proteins which nonetheless are fully functional and create no health problems at all for the individuals who have them.

Does It Run in the Family?

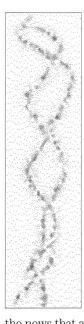

Chapter One

Introduction

The news is always a shock. No matter how caring the messenger or how gentle the words, the news that a family member has a "genetic" disorder pierces the family and delivers a stunning blow. Of course, hearing of any condition that can cause health problems or reduce one's life expectancy is bound to cause distress. But genetic or inherited disorders introduce additional, and sometimes difficult, concerns.

For Andrew and Donna Stone,* that terrible moment came shortly after the birth of their first child, Melissa. Within a few hours, their feelings of joy and exhilaration turned into fear and anxiety. Melissa had a serious problem, one that the doctors eventually diagnosed as a form of "spinal muscular atrophy" or SMA. The disorder causes nerves and muscles to deteriorate. It would shorten her life, causing her to die in infancy. And Melissa had inherited the condition from both of her parents. Over the next months, taking care of Melissa consumed all of Andrew and Donna's energy. Still they wondered: What does it mean that a disorder is inherited? There was no history of anyone on either

---

* All the names used are fictitious, and details of the cases have been changed to protect the privacy of the individuals and families involved.

side of the family having had this problem. So, where did this come from? Could they hope ever to have a healthy child? Was there any way to do a test to find out? If such a test did exist, could they afford to pay for it?

In the MacFarlane household, the unhappy moment came after five-year-old Arthur's prescreening session for the kindergarten class he was to enter in the fall. The teacher said that Arthur seemed to have very poor coordination. Harry and Jackie told her they had noticed that Arthur's physical progress was slow compared to that of his older sister. He was late in walking and had trouble climbing up the stairs to his room. They had even taken him to several doctors, including an orthopedic surgeon. Each time the experts assured them that Arthur would catch up. The teacher urged them to check into it once again. This time they consulted a neurologist who ordered blood tests. The blood tests suggested something was amiss. It seemed to take forever to arrange the follow-up studies and get back the reports. They all showed the same thing: Arthur had a disorder known as Duchenne muscular dystrophy.

Found only in boys, this form of muscular dystrophy is the result of a biological error that causes a slow but unrelenting breakdown of the muscles. This could have come about in either of two ways. The error could have first occurred in the single fertilized cell from which Arthur developed. Or it could have been passed on to him in the egg cell contributed by his mother. Not only did Harry and Jackie have to consider how best to care for their son in the years ahead, as the disorder intensified, but they were beset with other worries as well: Did Jackie have this flaw hidden in her other egg cells? Was it possible that their teenage daughter had inherited this same error? Though a girl having the flawed gene doesn't exhibit this disorder, it could show up in any son she might eventually have. Should their daughter be tested to find out if she has the flawed gene? Jackie's sister Jessie had married the previous year and was planning to have children of her own. Could Jessie's future children be at risk? Was there any need to let her—or their female cousins—know about this problem?

At a family wedding, a rare chance for the far-flung Tate family to get together, Phyllis Tate first got word that her eight-year-old niece, Meg, had been diagnosed half-a-year earlier with something called neurofibromatosis (or NF1). In its more severe forms, tumors begin to grow on nerves, interfering with body functions and causing life-threatening problems. Phyllis's dismay turned to terror when she learned that her brother-in-law, Meg's father, had also been found to have a mild form of NF1 and that her father-in-law, though he vigorously denied it, had the skin spots and tumors that often signal this disorder. Phyllis was three-months pregnant. Why hadn't her in-laws told her of this before she and Karl decided to start their own family? Was it possible that Karl also harbored whatever caused this problem? Was there any way to know if he did or if the fetus that was developing within her would be affected? Where could she could turn for information or advice?

The realization of potential serious health problems came more slowly for Sophie Baldwin. Gradually, one by one, the women on her mother's side of the family were falling victim to breast cancer. First it was a grandmother she hardly knew, then her aunt, then her cousin—the daughter of her mother's older brother—and then finally, her own mother! Something was traveling across the generations and was threatening to engulf her as well. What were her own chances of getting breast cancer? Did she dare to find out? Was there anything she could do if she did find out that her risk was high? Could the knowledge that she was destined to develop this cancer help her to make more realistic plans for her own life? Or could such knowledge be used against her, denying her job opportunities or health insurance?

The health problems these four families are facing are diverse, with some appearing in childhood, others not until the adult years; some affecting males, others females. The questions range from fears about prospects for children yet unborn to anxiety about other children already born as well as more distant family members, from concern about how to get needed information about themselves to worries about whether having that information (or sharing it with others) might introduce new difficulties. What these families have in common is that each of their problems originates, in part at least, within tiny units of heredity called *genes*. During reproduction, genes are passed along by egg and sperm cells. In the individuals mentioned above who are members of families with genetic disorders, one or more of their genes may not function properly and, as a result, could contribute to their own health problems or those of their children.

For millennia, humans have been fascinated by the obvious similarities between parents and children and have tried to understand how these similarities occur. The scientific study of inheritance, the field of genetics, was launched just at the start of the twentieth century. At first, this scientific work looked at general patterns of inheritance and used a set of basic rules to predict whether certain traits or features might be passed from parent to child. Over the succeeding decades, genetic study has progressed well beyond that early stage and has produced an impressive body of information on what genes actually are made of, how they are organized, and the ways in which they function or fail to function.

By the 1960s, some of this genetic knowledge was introduced into medical practice to help in making diagnoses and to provide the first tools for detecting the presence of some types of flawed genes in fetuses, children, and adults. Those first tests, though useful, were applicable only to a limited range of genetic disorders. They could not have answered the questions that the Stone, MacFarlane, Tate, or Baldwin families were asking. However, in recent years, dramatic new advances in genetics, biochemistry, and molecular biology have combined to create powerful tools for analyzing the genetic material. These tools have revolutionized and vastly expanded the opportunities for genetic testing, making it possible to obtain detailed genetic information on a scale unimaginable to the early geneticists. At the same time, the explosion of genetic information is raising new issues such as those troubling the families described here. In the pages that follow, we explore these new genetic tools and examine the spectrum of issues—personal and societal—surrounding decisions about whether or not to have a genetic test.

Chapter Two provides background information by explaining the basics of genetics and genetic testing and by defining the key terms. It surveys the types of genetic tests that are now available, beginning with early ones that gave the first hints about the human genetic makeup, and continuing to the newest kinds of tests—the DNA tests—that can uncover detailed information about the genetic material. In Chapter Three, the focus is on the practical aspects of obtaining genetic information. The central topics here include: how to find one's way to genetic information offered at genetic counseling centers in the medical community; what genetic counseling is and what it can and cannot provide; and how, once they get there, consumers can arrange to gain the most from their visit.

Specific types of genetic testing, the opportunities they offer, the burdens they might bring, and the dilemmas they produce are covered next. In Chapter Four, the emphasis is on tests for single genes whose presence is directly related to the onset of an illness at some point in a person's life. This is the kind of testing that Harry and Jackie MacFarlane could consider in trying to track the gene for Duchenne muscular dystrophy in their family, and that Donna and Andrew Stone could use in order to learn whether or not their next baby might have spinal muscular atrophy. Genes are shared among blood relatives in a family. Testing of one family member will alert other family members to the possibility that they may have inherited the same damaged gene. In fact, some forms of testing even require the participation of other members of the family.

Chapter Four draws from the families we have already met, as well as from dozens of other families who have contributed their experiences on the issues created by genetic testing. It also incorporates the views of clinicians, counselors, and caretakers. If any single message emerges from all these voices, it is that genetic tests can be of real value, but they are not right for everyone. Some will decide that they want to know their genetic status; others will postpone that journey or even decide never to set out on it. In making this decision, the combined experience of our interview group shows that four factors must be considered: the features of the disorder, the nature of the genetic test, the timing of the test, and the kinds of options that having the test information will bring.

It is always tempting to seek a guaranteed checklist that can provide an unerring guide to the correct decision, or to look to experts to tell us what to do. But what will be clear from the stories of people involved is that each situation is unique and that each decision has to be made on the basis of individual values, preferences, and circumstances. Each person is his or her own expert. Each person must determine which pathway is the best one to follow.

Chapter Five extends the examination of genetic testing to include the ways it can be used, and will increasingly be used, to predict susceptibility to disorders which result from the interaction of several different genes with environmental factors. Unlike the single-gene disorders of Chapter Four, the panorama of disorders which belong here tend to be the widespread, chronic health problems such as cancer, heart disease, diabetes, and the memory loss of Alzheimer's disease. Sophie Baldwin's questions about breast cancer will be raised by countless others at risk for cancer. Similar questions plague those concerned about the other chronic health problems. In Chapter Five, we find that the four factors central to decisions about testing for single-gene disorders are the very ones that should be considered when making personal decisions about testing for these more common illnesses. Here, too, we will see that individual circumstances differ markedly and that availability of genetic information does not determine whether it is useful or when it would be useful. No one set of rules and no single official policy is sufficient to serve as a definitive guide for the use of this type of genetic testing.

In the past, genetic information, even when incomplete and poorly understood, has been used to validate specific institutional and governmental policies. The twentieth century was witness to some of the most extreme human abuses carried out under the banner of "genetic improvement" and "purifying the gene pool." There are fears that the new forms of DNA testing, either for the presence of single genes that can bring on severe illnesses or for genes that can provide clues about susceptibility to chronic diseases, could be used (for their own purposes) by insurance companies, prospective employers, educational institutions, and even government agencies. In Chapter Six, we look at the social uses of genetic information from both a historical and a contemporary perspective. Current policies and proposed new policies are described. The somber historical record makes it prudent to build in a variety of safeguards to ward off abuse.

Additional factors can enter into decisions about genetic testing. Among these is the possibility that future improvements in testing procedures will provide more information than is available at present. Would this be a reason to postpone testing or to defer having children? Another element is the possibility that medical researchers might produce new kinds of treatments that will reduce or eliminate the adverse health consequences of some genetic disorders. One mode of treatment which is frequently anticipated is that of "gene therapy," that is, supplying people with the correct or functioning gene. Would this be a reason to go forward with having children? Chapter Seven examines the research track record in finding genes and in perfecting the genetic tests that look for miscues in those genes. It evaluates prospects for the development of treatments, including human gene therapy. This chapter also describes ways that consumers can help accelerate research efforts in areas of greatest interest to them.

Making informed decisions about genetic testing requires that accurate and up-to-date information be readily available. The medical community has established channels for communicating genetic information and for providing the services that accompany genetic testing. Professional geneticists serve on the front lines of information dispersal. However, it is clear from discussions with the consumer community that much of the genetic information people use as the basis for their decision-making is acquired informally—*outside the health-care system.* Most people get their information about the genetic basis of a disorder (and the kinds of tests and treatments available) not from the professional geneticists, but from other family members. Often what they learn through this "genetic grapevine" has been altered or misinterpreted or distorted as it is transmitted from person to person. Often, too, it is out of date, frozen in the moment of time at which the genetic disorder was first diagnosed. In Chapter Eight we will examine ways these informal networks can obtain and disperse accurate genetic information.

In the final chapter some suggestions are proposed for improvements in professional education, in genetic service delivery, and in support of the genetic grapevine.

In less than a century, genetics has changed remarkably. At first it was a field in which a few scientists pursued investigations hoping to find out something about the nature of abstract entities called genes. It is now a field in which many researchers use highly sophisticated techniques to gain a detailed view of our genetic inheritance. Medicine is also being transformed as clinicians are rapidly applying those findings to identify the genetic component of health problems. Genetic testing may soon be available on an unprecedented scale, presenting powerful opportunities and perplexing decisions for individuals and families.

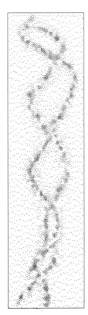

Chapter Two

Basics of Genetics and Genetic Testing

"Genes" come up in conversation all the time. We talk about genes when comparing ourselves with other members of our family. We notice similar physical features—Joey's eye color, the shape of Amanda's nose—and we automatically attribute them to genes. We go even further, ascribing our talents and abilities to genes. We say things like, "Joey got Nick's genes for fixing things and Amanda must have inherited my genes for good color sense." And we also blame genes for shortcomings. "All of the Blodgetts have always been extremely polite," we may tell a child who has misbehaved; "Those genes for your rude manners must have come from your father's side of the family!" From TV, movies, magazines, talk of genes comes at us from every corner of our culture. Regardless of whether genes play any part at all, it has become convenient to speak of them as being squarely at the center of our lives.

What genes really are and what they actually do is often quite different from what popular ideas suggest. This chapter will provide a basic introduction to genetics. The goal is not to turn the reader into a research scientist, but to show, with as few frills as possible, how it is that genes are sometimes connected with specific illnesses and how it is that genes may be passed on in a family from one generation to the next. In all of the later chapters, an effort has been made to include brief explanations of technical terms as they arise. This chapter provides more complete explanations. In particular, in this chapter we will see how scientists can test to find out if a person has a specific gene.

Genes Are Located on Chromosomes

Each of us possesses about fifty thousand to one hundred thousand different genes. (The exact number is not yet known.) All of these genes are repeated trillions of times throughout our body. *They are found in every one of our body's cells.* The *cell* is the building block that makes up all living organisms. Some organisms found in nature are amazingly small and relatively simple—only one cell in size. Humans, however, are very complex. The human body is composed of trillions of cells, almost all of them highly specialized into very different cell types such as muscle, nerve, blood, brain, and skin cells. These specialized cell types are arranged in larger groupings called organs and organ systems. All of these parts need to function in harmony if the whole body is to operate smoothly. To make this happen, a multitude of different tasks—involving growth, damage repair, and response to the environment—must be carried out successfully within each of the body's cells.

A gene is a unit which contains the instructions for how a cell should carry out a specific kind of task. Thus, a large number of genes is needed to supply all of the various instructions necessary for the vast array of tasks, or body functions, that characterize our living state. These genes are not floating about individually within each cell. They are connected together in long ribbon-like structures called *chromosomes.* Chromosomes are all stored in one portion of a cell, in a compartment called the *nucleus.*

Every species has a characteristic number of chromosomes. That number for corn is 20, for wheat, 42. In the frog the chromosome number is 26. In the mouse it is 40, and in the dog, 78. A photograph of the human chromosomes from a single cell can be seen in Figure 1. In

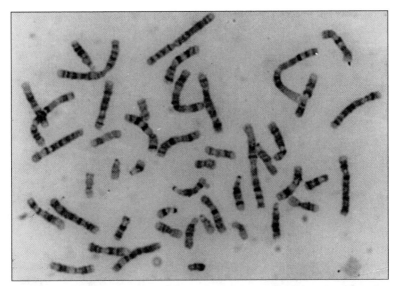

Figure 1. A photograph, taken through a microscope, showing the chromosomes present in a single human cell. *(Courtesy of Genetics and IVF Institute)*

Figure 2, these same chromosomes are arranged to form an organized picture, called a *karyotype.* In humans the chromosome number is 46. This full complement of 46 is made up of 23 pairs of chromosomes. The members of a pair are alike in size, shape, and the pattern of bands that appears after they are stained with a special dye in the laboratory.

Every human cell contains the same chromosome number, 46, except for two very special types of cells. Egg cells in women and sperm cells in men each contain 23 chromosomes. Each set of 23 contains one representative of every pair. When a sperm cell fuses with an egg cell in reproduction to begin the chain of events that can lead to a new individual, the standard human chromosome number of 46 is restored.

To help distinguish one pair from another, scientists numbered the pairs of chromosomes from 1 through 22. The chromosome pairs from 1 through 22 are called the *autosomes.* The *sex chromosomes* form the 23rd pair. This is the only pair in which the two members may be different. In females, the pair is comprised of two similar large-sized chromosomes which are not given a number but are identified by the

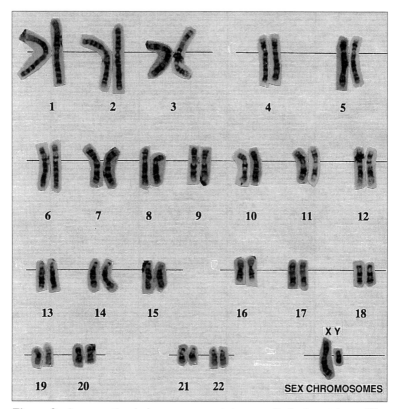

Figure 2. An organized chromosome picture, called a karyotype. The complete set of 46 chromosomes of Figure 1 has been arranged into the 23 matching pairs. At the lower right are the sex chromosomes. There is one X and one Y chromosome, showing that this individual is a male. A female has two X chromosomes. *(Courtesy of Genetics and IVF Institute)*

letter "X". In males, the sex chromosome pair has one X chromosome and a smaller chromosome, known as the "Y" chromosome, as the second member. Thus, for the sex chromosome pair, females are XX and males are XY.

All of the genes needed throughout the life span of an individual—from the fertilized egg to the adult—are filed away on the chromosomes. Because there are 23 pairs of human chromosomes, but tens of thousands of human genes, it is clear that each of the chromosomes we see in these photographs contains many many genes. Only the Y chromosome is gene poor. Current evidence suggests that the Y chromosome contains just a few genes.

Genes Are Made Up of DNA

Chromosomes are made up of one very special type of molecule called *DNA*. (The letters are a shorthand for the full chemical name of this substance: *d*eoxyribo*n*ucleic *a*cid.) Each chromosome is a very long thread of DNA. The reason we can see the chromosomes in the photographs is that the DNA they contain is very tightly coiled around itself. If the DNA in chromosome 1 were to be unwound like a ball of string and stretched to its full length, it would be a foot and a half long!

DNA is the genetic material. It is the chemical substance of which all genes are composed. The first glimpses into the structure of DNA came in 1953 and, by now, that structure has been examined in considerable detail. A sketch of the DNA molecule is shown in Figure 3. The molecule contains two strands which twist around each other in a spiral fashion, giving it the distinctive shape of a double helix.

The key parts of each DNA strand are chemical clusters of atoms; these atomic clusters are known as *bases.* There are just four types of bases in DNA. These are adenine (A), guanine (G), thymine (T), and cytosine (C). It is usual to refer to each of these bases just by its initial. Between each base on one strand and the corresponding base on the opposite strand, there is a chemical connection. These chemical connections (or bonds) hold the two strands together and give stability to the whole DNA molecule. These connections are particular in that an A base in one strand forms a bond only with a T in the opposite strand, and a G bonds only with a C.

A gene is a section of DNA along the chromosome. That section has a definite beginning and a definite end. The section of DNA which constitutes a gene possesses a specific *sequence of bases* which is a code that determines the specific function that the gene controls. (These functions are discussed further in the next few pages.) Genes vary in size. Some are small, occupying a very short section of the DNA.

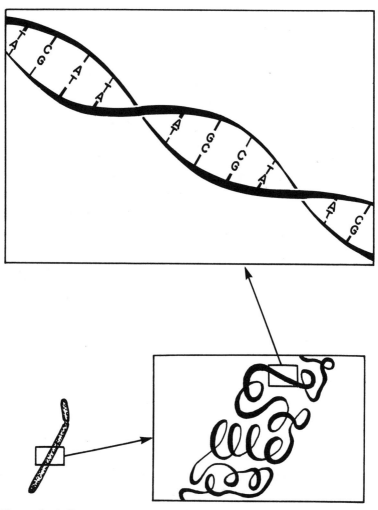

Figure 3. A diagram representing magnified views of a chromosome's structure. The chromosome is at the lower left. A magnified portion of the chromosome (the section in the small rectangle) reveals that it consists of a long thread, the DNA molecule (shown at the lower right). A magnified portion of the DNA molecule shows that the thread consists of two strands that are held together by A-T and G-C bonds. The two strands twist around each other in a double helix.

Others are huge, extending a considerable distance along the DNA. We can imagine each of the chromosomes as a cookbook containing hundreds or even thousands of individual recipes (some brief, some lengthy), all bound together, one following the next. In a cookbook, recipes of the same kind—appetizers, salads, meat dishes, desserts—each have their own separate chapter. But on a chromosome, the genetic information is largely a jumble of different types of instructions for different types of tasks. The gene that helps a muscle contract may be positioned on the chromosome immediately following the gene responsible for the early development of the digestive system and immediately preceding one of the genes involved in producing eye color.

And unlike a cookbook that has no (or very few) blank pages, each chromosome contains vast stretches of DNA that do not seem to have any function. Some scientists call these regions "junk" DNA, and there are estimates that about 90 percent of human DNA may be of this type. Areas of so-called junk DNA may contain relics of genes from our evolutionary past, antique recipes for functions that are no longer required by us. These regions may also contain the remains of viruses which infected our ancestors in eons past and inserted their tiny bits of genetic material into chromosomes where they now lie abandoned.

Genes Work by Producing Proteins

How can a gene, which is just a length of DNA along a chromosome, affect the activities of an organism? It can do this because the specific order, or sequence, of the bases (the A's, G's, T's, and C's) on one strand provides the recipe or code for making a specific *protein.* Proteins are cell molecules which are composed of smaller units (called amino acids) connected together in a linear fashion. Within the nucleus of the cell, where the DNA resides, a complex set of operations occurs. The instructions provided by the sequence of bases (found in the gene along one DNA strand) allow a corresponding sequence of amino acids to be assembled into a protein molecule. In this way, each gene is responsible for producing a specific protein.

Most of the life-supporting work of living organisms is carried out by proteins. There are several different kinds of proteins with different types of functions. *Enzyme proteins* (better known just as "enzymes") act as catalysts, speeding up chemical reactions and thus allowing critical life functions—digestion, growth, excretion, and response to the environment—to take place rapidly and efficiently. *Structural proteins* are responsible for forming the various parts of our body's architecture. The many different types of components that we can see (such as bones, hair, and nails) which shape and give support to our bodies, as well as ones that can be seen only with the aid of a microscope (such as the membranes surrounding cells or the small particles found within cells) contain proteins. *Regulatory proteins* help coordinate different chemical processes that need to occur in a synchronized way. Proteins are central in all the activities necessary for life.

We need to remember that proteins are produced under the direction of specific genes. And proteins (for example, the enzyme proteins) are specialized to carry out particular functions. Even though every cell of an individual has all of the same genes, the array of proteins produced in different types of cells is *not* the same. Each type of cell—whether it is from a muscle, nerve, skin, liver, and so on—results from the production of a different mix of proteins. So in muscle cells, proteins are produced that are necessary for the muscle to contract. But a muscle cell does not produce proteins involved in vision. Red blood cells produce those proteins necessary to transport oxygen around the body, but they don't produce any of the proteins involved in muscle contraction. Our body cells, with their multitude of different proteins, provide the framework that makes life possible.

Genes (Nearly Always) Come in Pairs

Chromosomes in a pair (for instance, the two chromosomes in the chromosome 9 pair) contain the same arrangement of genes. Suppose a gene for a particular enzyme occurs at a certain position along the DNA molecule of one chromosome of the pair. The gene for that same enzyme will be found on the other chromosome at exactly the same position along *its* DNA molecule. We say that this gene occurs at the same location, or *locus,* on both members of the chromosome pair. This means that there are two genes for every specific function or task that must be carried out. The only exception to this rule is in the XY sex-chromosome pair in males. The X and Y chromosomes differ greatly in their gene content. The X chromosome contains many genes for many different types of activities. The Y chromosome has very few genes, and the genes it does have seem to be only the ones responsible for triggering the formation of the male reproductive system during the early development of the embryo. As a result, males have only one copy of each gene that is located on the X chromosome. Females, because their sex chromosome pair contains two X chromosomes, have two copies.

Members of a Pair of Genes Can Differ from Each Other

The two genes at the same locus (one on each chromosome in the chromosome pair) can be identical. That is, they can both have precisely the same sequence of bases along the length of DNA corresponding to the genes. When this occurs, both genes provide identical information for their particular protein product. However, the two genes do not have to be exactly the same, and very often they are not. Genes at the same locus can possess somewhat different DNA sequences. And one change in the DNA sequence may result in a change in the protein made by the cell, in the same way that a change in one ingredient of a recipe may result in a change in the dish made by the cook.

The information contained in the DNA can be altered in many different ways. Consider a short sequence of bases (. . . TAGACAT . . .) on one strand. Suppose that this is a part of a much longer sequence within a gene. If one or more of the bases is missing (. . . TAGACT . . . or . . . TAGAT . . .), sequence information will be left out. If the opposite occurs (. . . TAGACAAAAT . . .), extra base sequence information will be present. Sometimes, a group of three bases may come to be repeated over and over again (. . . TAGACATCATCATCATCAT . . .).

Sometimes the total number of bases is the same but one DNA base has been substituted for another (. . . GAGACAT . . .). In all of these cases, the instructions (the protein recipe) provided by the gene have been changed.

Any permanent change or alteration in the base sequence of a gene is called a *mutation.* Mutations can arise at the time that the sperm cells and egg cells needed for reproduction are forming. During the formation of these reproductive cells (or *gametes*), chromosomes make more copies of themselves by doubling. When chromosomes double, each of the 46 chromosomes splits down the center of the DNA molecule. The double helix unzips to yield two separate single strands. Each single strand then forms a whole new second strand by collecting DNA bases floating about in the cell and assembling them alongside. Each base in the original strand joins to one in the newly forming strand following the rule that A's join to T's and that G's join to C's. This is a huge task. About three billion new bases must be correctly positioned. There are enzymes whose job it is to fix those spots where mismatches have occurred. Even so, errors in the final sequence can still creep in during this critical period in which new DNA is being made. Mutations can also arise in chromosomes at other times, when outside agents (such as ultraviolet radiation from the sun, X-rays from medical tests, or chemicals in the environment) cause the DNA to become altered in some way.

Mutations in a gene can alter its protein product. Some variations in the gene's base sequence have minor effects. The protein produced may be slightly altered, but still function perfectly well. But other changes can have a big impact. The protein may carry out its allotted function poorly. Or the sequence change may prevent the protein from being made at all. Genetic disorders are the result of the presence of such mutations.

Single-gene disorders come about when one or both of the members of a *gene pair* are unable to do their job properly. Even if all the other tens of thousands of genes are doing their jobs perfectly well, the error at just one gene pair may throw a monkey wrench into the way the body functions. This brings on health problems that can, on occasion, be extremely serious, even life threatening. Disorders such as spinal muscular atrophy, Duchenne muscular dystrophy, sickle-cell anemia, neurofibromatosis, and about five thousand others are currently known to fall into this category. (Patterns of inheritance for single-gene disorders are discussed below. Single-gene disorders are also discussed in Chapter Four.)

Multifactorial or *complex disorders* come about when genetic and environmental factors interact in a complicated way, which is still poorly understood. For such disorders, it appears that not just one gene pair but several different gene pairs are unable to function properly. There is also a strong connection to features of the environment, such as diet, smoking habits, or exposure to things like radiation, chemicals, and infections. Cancer, heart disease, diabetes, and many other common health problems fall into this category. (This type of disorder is discussed in Chapter Five.)

Single-Gene Disorders Show Different Patterns of Inheritance

No one has a perfect collection of genes. All of us have some mutations in our DNA. It is estimated that each of us has about eight genes where changes have occurred that could severely impair our health. Fortunately, a change in our DNA does not always show up as a genetic disorder. Whether or not a genetic disorder actually occurs depends on where the gene is located, what type of task it directs, and how well the other genes that are present function.

People have long sought ways to make sense of the patterns of inheritance they were observing in their families. With the groundbreaking experiments of the nineteenth-century Austrian monk, Gregor Mendel (whose work was rediscovered in 1900), and innumerable other studies carried out around the world since that time, it has been possible to identify several different patterns of inheritance exhibited by single genes. These patterns make it possible to understand how disorders can be passed through generations. Though our emphasis here is on genetic disorders, it is important to keep in mind that these same patterns underlie the inheritance of other human traits, such as hair type and blood type.

THE AUTOSOMAL DOMINANT PATTERN

A *dominant mutation* is one that shows up in the form of a noticeable health problem even when only one gene of the pair has the mutation. If the dominant mutation has occurred within a gene located on one of the 22 pairs of autosomes, it is called an *autosomal dominant* mutation. Huntington disease (affecting brain cells), neurofibromatosis (affecting the growth of nerve cells), and some forms of retinitis pigmentosa (affecting vision) are examples of disorders brought on by autosomal dominant mutations.

Let us suppose that there is a gene that provides the instructions for a protein destined to become part of our bone structure. Both members of the gene pair direct the formation of that bone-structure protein. However, the mutated gene's instructions create a protein that is defective. The cell or body structure that is assembled from these two different protein products could have much altered properties. Imagine what would happen if you built a wall with a mixed supply of bricks, half of which were much smaller and weaker than standard bricks. The wall would look different and be weaker than one made entirely of standard bricks. In the same way, if one member of the gene pair guides the formation of impaired bone-structure protein, the result can be weakened bones throughout the body, even if the other gene guides the formation of the standard protein product.

An autosomal dominant mutant gene can show up in several generations of a family. Figure 4 shows how this is possible. An affected individual is one who has both a mutant gene and a standard— or "normal"—gene. Such an individual will produce two different types of eggs (if female) or sperm (if male). Half of the eggs or sperm will have a set of 23 chromosomes that includes the chromosome with the normal gene; half of the eggs or sperm will have a set of 23 chromosomes that includes the chromosome with the mutant gene. Half of the time, a fertilized egg produced at conception will receive (by chance) the normal gene. Half of the time, a fertilized egg will receive

Autosomal Dominant Inheritance Pattern

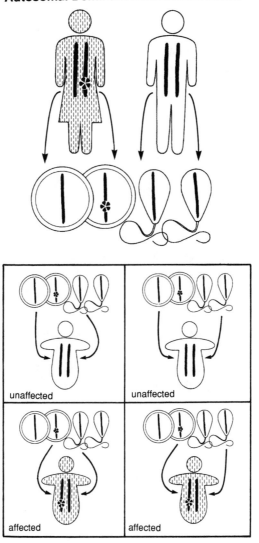

Figure 4. *Autosomal dominant inheritance pattern.* Here the mother is affected (shown patterned); she has the mutant gene (shown as an asterisk). Of the four possible combinations of sperm and egg, two contain the mutant gene. The chance of a child being affected, at each pregnancy, is 50 percent.

(by chance) the mutant gene. A dominant mutant gene has a 50 percent chance of being passed from parent to child, where its presence will be evident. In the case of autosomal dominant disorders, males and females have an equal chance of being affected. In general, unaffected individuals have no defective genes to pass on and so this type of disorder cannot show up in their children.

A NOTE ON PROBABILITY

In small families, one cannot expect to see displayed all of these features of the autosomal dominant inheritance pattern. The 50 percent chance of any particular child being affected is, it must be emphasized, a *probability*. It means that if 1,000 families in this situation (one parent with an autosomal dominant gene) have 2,000 children, then about 1,000 of the children will be affected. But, it can happen, in a specific family with two or three children, that all of the children are affected. It can also happen that none are affected. It can happen that affected individuals in one family are all males, or all females. Each fusion of sperm and egg is a separate, independent, chance event. The joining together of parental genes is completely independent of whatever may have occurred before in the family. Having one unaffected child (or one affected child) does *not* change the odds for the next child. The probability remains 50 percent.

The rule to remember is this: *The odds are the same at each pregnancy.* Another example of this rule is described at the end of the next section.

THE AUTOSOMAL RECESSIVE PATTERN

In contrast to dominant mutations, a *recessive* mutation is one that shows up (as a noticeable health problem) only when *both* genes of the pair have the mutation. As before, if the recessive mutation has occurred within a gene located on one of the 22 pairs of autosomes, it is called an *autosomal recessive* mutation. Examples of such mutations are those that lead to sickle-cell anemia (affecting red blood cells), cystic fibrosis (affecting mucous thickness), and spinal muscular atrophy.

Let us suppose here that we are looking at a gene pair which contains the instructions for making an enzyme. This may be an enzyme responsible for breaking down a toxic substance that, unless it is removed, can poison a cell. If an individual has one normal gene with instructions for making a functional enzyme and one mutant recessive gene which leads to an impaired enzyme, there will be no health problems related to that enzyme. The amount of enzyme produced under the direction of the one functional gene is sufficient to ensure that all the toxic substance is removed. This means that even one gene providing correct information yields enough normal protein for each cell to carry out that task adequately. A healthy person like this, who has one normal gene and one mutant gene, is called a *carrier. It is important to emphasize that carriers are healthy. Carriers do not suffer any ill effects of having the recessive mutant gene.* In fact, most carriers do not have any idea that they have the mutant gene. We *all* carry several recessive mutant genes. We don't know about them, usually because each is masked by the presence of a normal gene on the other chromosome.

Recessive mutant genes *may* lead to disorders in children whose parents are *both* carriers (see Figure 5). When both parents are carriers, it is possible for two mutant genes, one contributed by each parent, to come together when an egg is fertilized. Each carrier parent produces two types of egg or sperm. One type will have the chromosome with the normal gene; the other will have the mutant gene. When both parents are carriers, there is one chance in four that an egg and a sperm each containing the same mutant gene will join with one another to form the fertilized egg. When that happens, both genes of the pair will be mutant genes. All the enzyme protein that is produced by those mutant genes will be defective. With only defective protein present, a vital cell process, such as the removal of the toxic substance, will not occur. The health of individual cells and of the person with these genes will be impaired. As we see in Figure 5, carrier parents can also have children who are carriers like themselves, and they can also have children who do not have the mutant gene at all. At each pregnancy, the probability is 25 percent for having a child with a disorder, 50 percent for having a healthy child who is a carrier, and 25 percent for having a healthy child who is not a carrier.

Autosomal Recessive Inheritance Pattern

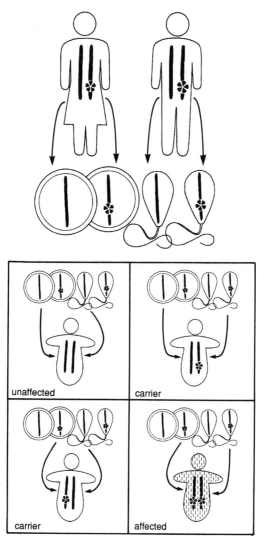

Figure 5. *Autosomal recessive inheritance pattern.* Here each parent is healthy and is a carrier, having one normal and one mutant gene (shown as an asterisk). Each parent is unaffected because the normal gene masks the recessive mutant gene. Of the four possible combinations of sperm and egg, one contains no mutant gene (unaffected noncarrier), two contain one mutant gene (unaffected carrier, like each parent), and one contains two mutant genes (affected, shown patterned). The chance of a child having the disorder is 25 percent.

Because its presence is masked by a functionally normal gene, an autosomal recessive mutant gene can remain hidden for many generations. It is only when both partners have the same recessive mutant gene that there is a 25 percent chance, with each pregnancy, that the disorder will show up. For this reason, genetic disorders brought on by autosomal recessive genes tend to appear unexpectedly. Often, no one in the family can recall any illness like it having occurred before. When an illness does occur, this is a signal that other siblings in the same family may be carriers, as may be cousins, aunts, uncles, and grandparents. For autosomal recessive disorders, males and females are equally likely to be affected.

As I've stressed, it should *not* be expected that any particular family will have a distribution of inheritance that is the same as the average distribution of 25 percent/50 percent/25 percent. There is no "requirement" that one child in a family of four has to be affected. There is no guarantee that already having one affected child means that the next three will be unaffected. And it is not true that having several unaffected children means that the next child is "due" to be affected. Sometimes more than one child in a family may inherit the double-recessive combination. Sometimes, none of them will. Geneticists are fond of saying that "chance has no memory." This is their way of reminding people that the odds two carrier parents face stay the same at every new pregnancy.

THE X-LINKED PATTERN OF INHERITANCE

The sex chromosome pair introduces some changes into the standard patterns of inheritance we have been examining. All genes that are on the X chromosome are said to be X-linked. Body cells of males have only one X chromosome. The other chromosome of their sex chromosome pair, the Y, has its own few unique genes. Thus, males have only one copy of each of their X-linked genes. For all of these genes, one copy is enough to provide sufficient amounts of protein to meet cell needs. However, if a gene on the X chromosome of a male contains a mutation, there will be no second copy of the gene to rely on. There is no corresponding gene on the Y chromosome that can mask it. This means that the trait or disorder associated with the mutant gene will show up. For example, if there is a mutation in the X-chromosome gene which contains the instructions for making a certain muscle protein called dystrophin, it will show up as Duchenne muscular dystrophy, a disorder in which muscles deteriorate. If there is a mutation in the gene which contains the instructions for making a protein required for blood to clot when there is an injury, it will show up as hemophilia. Females who are carriers of these flawed genes generally show no sign of the disorder. They have, as part of their sex chromosome pair, a second X chromosome with a functional gene. This means that X-linked recessive mutations show up more commonly in males.

Males always receive the X-chromosome member of their sex chromosome pair from their mothers. They always get their Y chromosome, which confers their maleness, from their fathers. Because males inherit their X chromosome from their mothers, the pattern of inheritance of X-linked recessive mutations differs from that for autosomal recessive mutations. A woman who is a carrier will produce two different types of eggs; half will have the X chromosome with the normal gene, half will have the X chromosome containing the mutant gene. If an egg cell containing the mutant gene is fertilized by a sperm cell bearing a Y chromosome, there will be no way to mask the presence of the mutant gene and its effects will be seen in that male child. If that egg cell with the mutant gene is fertilized by a sperm cell with an X chromosome (and with the normal gene), the resulting healthy female child will be a carrier like her mother.

As seen in Figure 6, on average, *X-linked recessive* disorders will be expected to appear in half of the male offspring of a woman who is a carrier. The other half, those males who had received from her the X chromosome with the functional gene, will be unaffected. (Each pregnancy, of course, is a new toss of the genetic dice that is not influenced by what has happened before in the family.) Of her daughters, on average, half will be expected to be carriers like herself and half will have received two copies of the normal gene. None of these females will have the disorder. When X-linked recessive mutant genes show up in males in two or more different places in a family, the affected

X-Linked Recessive Inheritance Pattern

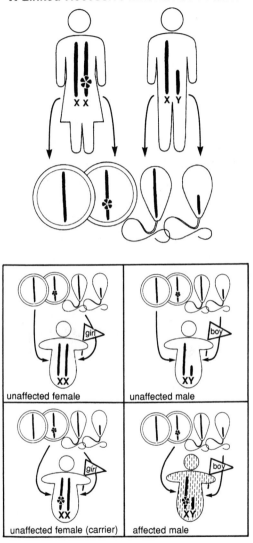

Figure 6. *X-linked recessive inheritance pattern.* One of the mother's X chromosomes contains the mutant gene. All the daughters (XX) will be healthy, although half of them will be carriers (like their mother). But each son (XY) has a 50 percent chance of developing the disorder, because each has a 50 percent chance of inheriting the mother's mutant gene and there is no corresponding gene on the Y chromosome to mask it.

relatives are all related to each other by females who are carriers. X-linked recessive disorders can also appear to "skip" one or several generations, as the gene is passed down through females who are carriers of the recessive mutation. The only way a female can be affected is if her father has an X-linked recessive disorder and her mother is a carrier of a mutation in that very same gene. This can happen when an X-linked mutation occurs at a fairly high frequency in the population, as is the case for the mutation that leads to colorblindness.

X-linked dominant mutations are very rare. When they occur, they show up in both males and females. If a man has a disorder brought on by such a mutation, all his daughters (who must have inherited his X chromosome to develop as females) will have the disorder. All of his sons (who must have inherited his Y chromosome) will be unaffected. If a female has an X-linked dominant mutation, there is a 50 percent chance of each of her children, sons and daughters, being affected.

Frequently, an X-linked disorder appears in a family in which there is no previous history of the disorder. Its sudden appearance can be explained in one of two ways. The mutant gene may have been present for generations, passed along by carrier females who were completely unaware of its presence. By chance, the chromosome bearing the mutant gene had never been paired with a Y chromosome. Or it may be that a new mutation has occurred. Geneticists have estimated that one in three new cases of an X-linked disorder are the result of a new mutation. In the case of a new mutation, the mother of the affected boy is not a carrier.

It Has Become Possible to Test for Genetic Illness

Today the study of human genes is one of the most active areas in all of medical research. Scientists have developed many different procedures for examining the genetic material. These procedures are revealing a great deal about how changes in the genetic material can lead to various kinds of health problems. Once the relationship is understood, genetic tests that look for such changes become possible. The first forms of human genetic testing, initiated several decades ago and still widely used today, rely on two types of laboratory techniques: *microscope-based techniques* that examine the chromosomes, and *biochemical techniques* that examine the actual protein components that are present.

The microscope-based techniques make it possible to view all of a cell's chromosomes (just as we have already seen in Figures 1 and 2). These techniques provide a picture which reveals the total chromosome number and the overall arrangement of the chromosomal material. An incorrect number of chromosomes (above or below the normal total of 46) or an incorrect arrangement of the chromosomal material (such as the loss of part of a chromosome) can be at the root of some disorders. Best known among these is Down syndrome, a form of mental retardation which occurs when a mistake in the formation of eggs or sperm leaves an additional chromosome in the fertilized egg. Individuals who have Down syndrome have an extra chromosome 21 (giving them three chromosome 21s instead of two). They therefore have 47, instead of 46, chromosomes in total.

Biochemical techniques give information about the status of individual genes. These techniques measure the amount of protein that has been produced by the pair of genes responsible for that protein. The amount of functional protein present indicates whether or not any mutant genes are present. For instance, the absence of one enzyme protein (officially hexosaminidase A, but called "hex-A" for short) causes the multiple and injurious features of Tay-Sachs disease, a lethal autosomal recessive genetic disorder. Affected babies have inherited two defective copies of the gene for this protein and produce no functional enzyme. They die in early childhood. Carriers, those individuals with one normal and one defective gene, produce only half as much of the enzyme. This amount still provides more than enough functional protein to protect them, so they have no adverse health effects. Biochemical tests that reveal a reduced level of the hex-A enzyme allow the carriers, who otherwise have no symptoms of any sort, to be identified and distinguished from noncarriers, those who possess two functional genes and produce high levels of the enzyme.

In some genetic disorders, the protein is produced, but it has altered properties because of a mutation in the gene that produces it. The presence of such proteins with altered properties can also be picked up through the use of biochemical procedures. Some examples of the disorders that can be detected are those involving the hemoglobin molecule, which transports oxygen throughout the body, or the collagen molecule, which provides structural support throughout the body.

The development of microscope-based techniques for looking at chromosomes, and of biochemical techniques for examining proteins, ushered in the new era of genetic medicine. Genetic testing of people, from babies to adults, could now be readily accomplished by taking a sample of blood. For example, the white blood cells in the sample could be treated in the laboratory to make the chromosomes visible, allowing them to be examined (as in Figure 2). The red blood cells could be biochemically tested to see what kind of hemoglobin is present.

Testing of the fetus, prior to birth, is possible using procedures which collect fetal cells. In one of these procedures, called *amniocentesis,* a sample of the amniotic fluid (the fluid surrounding the fetus) is collected. The fluid is drawn out using a needle inserted through the mother's abdominal wall and uterus and into the amniotic sac. This procedure is done at about the sixteenth week of gestation. The amniotic fluid contains fetal cells whose chromosome makeup and protein makeup can be examined. In another of these procedures, *chorionic villus sampling,* cells on the outside of the chorionic sac (the outermost covering surrounding the fetus) are collected at about the ninth week of gestation. Both means of gathering cells carry with them a very small risk of problems that may terminate the pregnancy.

Newer Genetic Tests—DNA Tests—Are Even More Powerful

For the vast majority of genetic disorders, the microscope and biochemical tests are of no use at all. Most genetic disorders result from defects in a single gene. We cannot see the features of a single, tiny gene by just looking at a picture of the entire chromosome. Moreover, it is often the case that we simply do not yet know the specific protein whose absence or alteration (due to the altered gene) is associated with a genetic disorder. When there is no identified protein to seek out, it is not possible to carry out biochemical measurements to determine how much total protein is present or whether that protein is changed in any way. Even when the protein (for which the gene codes) is known, in order to study it biochemically in a prenatal test, that protein must be made by the cells that we are able to collect—the amniotic fluid cells. It does no good to look for a protein like hemoglobin in amniotic fluid cells, since these cells do not manufacture hemoglobin.

Laboratory techniques developed in recent years now make it possible to go beyond looking at whole chromosomes or measuring the protein products of specific genes. There are techniques that can identify the chromosome on which a gene is located, and that can pinpoint the position of the gene on that chromosome (more on this in Chapter Seven). The newest techniques examine the DNA itself. They are capable of locking onto specific places in or near the DNA of a gene and of checking out certain features of that DNA. These new capabilities in laboratory techniques have led to revolutionary changes in genetic testing. Several new types of tests are now possible.

THE DIRECT TEST

A *direct test* can recognize tiny alterations or mutations that actually change the instructions contained in the DNA of a gene. These are the very changes that damage the gene's ability to produce a protein the organism needs. The loss of a very small region of a gene, even a region as small as a single base pair, can be detected. Changes in the DNA sequence of the gene—even by one base pair—can be spotted. If repeated sequences of bases occur, the number of such *repeats* can be counted. Thus direct DNA tests disclose precise details of a gene's DNA.

The power of these direct DNA tests to reveal the status of genes is extraordinary. But there are limits. A direct DNA test can be done only when we know the specific gene involved in the genetic disorder. And not only must we know the gene, but we must also know what specific flaws within the DNA of that gene cause it to malfunction. For instance, direct tests can be done to see if the single mutation responsible for sickle-cell anemia is present. However, a test cannot be done if the gene has been identified but each family possesses its own unique mutation—a *private mutation*—as in neurofibromatosis and some types of hemophilia. The value of the direct test is diminished if the gene is a very long one and there are so many different possible mutations within it that it is not possible or practical to test for each and every one. In such a case, the direct test can be designed to look for the most common mutations, but not the rare or unusual ones. Direct tests for Duchenne muscular dystrophy can pick up 60 percent of the mutations; for cystic fibrosis, 90 percent of the mutations can be found. This means that many people with these disorders will have mutations that the test cannot detect.

THE LINKAGE TEST

There is another approach to genetic testing. It allows a prediction to be made about the presence of a mutated gene even if there is, at present, no clue at all about what the gene itself is, what changes have occurred in its DNA sequence, or what function the gene serves in the cells. This approach is the *linkage test.* Linkage tests can often be used in situations in which a direct DNA test cannot be done.

What happens in a linkage test is this: When there is no way to detect the "target" gene directly (to determine whether the flawed form of that gene has been inherited), a known region of DNA located *close* to the target gene can be used as a "marker" for the target gene. By following the marker, predictions about the actual state of the nearby target gene can be made. The marker serves as an indicator in much the same way that the tall flag attached to a child's bicycle alerts a motorist to the presence of the child, who might be hidden from view by cars, bushes, or signs as she pedals along. Similarly, a buoy floating on the surface of the water warns sailors of a hidden hazard located below the surface.

Linkage testing relies on the strong tendency of two regions of DNA that are near each other, linked together on a chromosome, to stay together when the sperm and egg cells (which contain 23 chromosomes, one from each pair) are formed. The closer these two DNA regions are to each other on the chromosome, the more likely it is they will stay together and be inherited together. The farther apart they are, the less likely it is that they will stay together. If the marker and the target gene are not very close, they can occasionally become separated from each other by the processes of chromosome breakage and exchange of pieces which occurs between members of the same chromosome pair during egg and sperm formation. Such reshuffling of DNA regions is a normal event.

Several types of DNA markers are useful for linkage testing. One type of marker can simply be another gene which is located very close to the target gene and which produces a protein that can be measured. In Figure 7-a, we see that a mutant gene that we cannot otherwise detect is linked with a gene at a nearby locus whose distinctive protein product *can* be detected. Keeping track of the marker gene (through its protein product) provides an important clue about whether or not the mutant gene has been inherited. If we find that the marker gene has been passed along from parent to child, it is a strong indication that the nearby mutant gene has also been inherited. Conversely, the absence of the marker gene is a strong indication that the mutant gene is also absent.

An even more useful kind of marker takes advantage of differences in base sequence of the DNA molecule in the vicinity of the target gene. Tiny variations in the base sequence occur at many places scattered throughout the DNA. By some estimates, a single base-pair variation along the DNA molecule occurs about once every five hundred base pairs. This means that the DNA sequence found on one chromosome can and does differ slightly from the DNA sequence of its partner chromosome. The DNA molecules of the partner chromosomes can also differ from each other in another way: Some places on the chromosomes can contain extended sequences where one type of base alternates with another many times. For example, there are places where C's alternate with A's. One chromosome of a pair may have very few of these C-A repeats (perhaps six), while the other chromosome may have a large

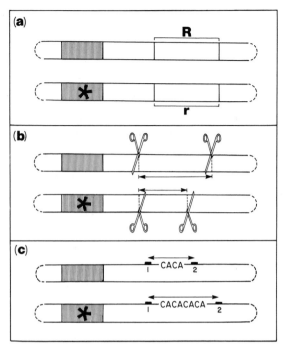

Figure 7. *Three types of linkage testing.* Linkage testing is used when a direct test for the mutant gene can't be done. A linkage test provides an estimate of the probability that the mutant gene (shown by the asterisk) has been passed on to the child. In each case described here, the chromosome pair shown is from the parent with the mutant gene. The child's DNA (not shown in this figure) is tested and compared to the DNA of this parent.

In (a), another gene ("r"), known to be a close neighbor of the mutant gene, is tracked. If this marker gene is found in the child's DNA, then there is a high probability that the mutant gene has been inherited.

In (b), restriction enzymes (the scissors) are used to cut the DNA molecule wherever a certain base sequence occurs. Such a sequence can occur at different locations on partner chromosomes (as indicated by the scissor positions at the right). When this happens, different-length fragments are produced by the action of these enzymes. In the case shown here, the short fragment is the marker for the mutant gene. If the short fragment is found in the child's DNA, then there is a high probability that the mutant gene has been inherited.

In (c), a technique is used (PCR) that copies sections between two specific end points (labeled 1 and 2) on the DNA molecule. In the case shown here, the DNA between the end points is longer (has more C-A repeats) near the mutant gene and shorter (fewer C-A repeats) near the normal gene. So here the occurrence of the longer copies (in a PCR test of the child's DNA) is the marker for a high probability of the presence of the mutant gene.

number of C-A repeats (perhaps thirty) at the very same location. These variations are generally without any harmful effects and go unnoticed by the organism, since the vast majority of them occur in those extensive "junk" DNA portions of the chromosomes, which were mentioned earlier.

While of little or no consequence to the life of the cell, these small changes in the DNA can be pressed into service as linked markers. This is because they provide a means for breaking the long threads of chromosomal DNA into different-sized pieces in the region of the target gene. There is a special kind of enzyme, called a *restriction enzyme,* which acts by roaming over the chromosomal DNA and breaking the DNA molecule wherever a particular sequence of bases (such as GAATTC) appears on one of the two strands. In the laboratory, restriction enzymes are introduced into a sample of an individual's DNA. As a result of the action of these restriction enzymes, the long DNA molecules forming each chromosome break up into many shorter lengths or fragments. Partner chromosomes usually break apart in the same places and produce fragments of the same size. But, as we see in Figure 7-b, it can happen that the sequence that causes a break is present on one chromosome of the pair, but is absent at the equivalent site on the other chromosome. When this situation occurs, the breaking-apart action of the restriction enzyme yields DNA fragments of different lengths in this region of each chromosome, indicating there are differences in the sequences.

Fragments of different lengths can also be generated if the chromosomes have different numbers of C-A repeats (or some other short repeats) in the same region of the two chromosomes (see Figure 7-c). The technique which produces these fragments is called the *polymerase chain reaction* (PCR). With this technique, short stretches of DNA between two fixed points on the DNA molecule are copied over and over again. The length of the copies that are produced depends on the number of C-A repeats *between* the two fixed points.

Sophisticated laboratory methods have been developed to find out when fragments of different lengths have been produced. This allows target genes to be followed by their association with particular-sized fragments produced after restriction enzyme or PCR treatment. In this form of DNA testing, it is simply the length of a DNA fragment (in the region of the chromosome near the target gene) which provides the key to figuring out whether or not the normal or the mutant gene has been inherited.

Linkage testing is more complicated than direct DNA testing because it first must be determined which markers are adjacent to the target genes on both chromosomes. The nature of the markers found on the chromosomes differs from family to family. Several family members, most especially those members who have the genetic disorder in question, need to be tested to figure out which marker is traveling along with the mutant gene and which with the normal gene. It is also necessary that the marker which travels along with the mutant gene be different from the marker that travels along with the normal gene. If the two markers are identical, then there will be no way to distinguish the mutant from the normal gene.

Therefore, linkage testing will only yield information about which versions of the gene are present when the marker relationships are known and when there are differences between markers linked to mutant genes and markers linked to normal genes. Even when all these conditions are met, one has to be cautious when drawing conclusions from the results. What is really happening in linkage testing is the making of informed guesses (or predictions) based on a region of DNA at a short distance from the actual target gene. Remember that regions of DNA can sometimes be exchanged between chromosomes; therefore it can occasionally happen that the markers have been switched. (The farther apart they are, the more opportunity there is for switching to occur.) The marker originally linked with the mutant gene will now be attached to the normal gene and vice versa.

Thus, linkage testing cannot give an absolutely certain answer about whether a particular gene is present. What it can provide is the likelihood or *probability* that a particular form of a gene has been inherited along with its marker. A typical result of a genetic test for an autosomal dominant mutation might be stated in this way: "There is a 95 percent chance that you have inherited the normal form of a gene from an affected parent and a 5 percent chance that you have inherited the mutant gene." Many genetic counselors prefer to present the results as "high-risk" or "low-risk" so that it is clear that some uncertainty remains.

THE EXCLUSION TEST

Linkage testing has occasionally been used even though a direct test for a mutant gene may be available. The reason for performing the linkage test might be as follows: A person who has a 50 percent chance of having inherited a gene for a late-onset disorder may want to gain some information about the genetic status of a fetus while still remaining ignorant of his or her own actual status. When this is desired, a "nondisclosing" linkage test—also called an *exclusion test*—is used. In an exclusion test, DNA markers from the fetus are compared with the markers of the affected grandparent (the one, say, with Huntington disease) and the healthy grandparent. If a DNA marker from the affected grandparent is found in the fetal cells, then the fetus, like the parent, has a 50 percent chance of having inherited the mutant gene. If, instead, a DNA marker from the healthy grandparent is found, then it is very likely that the fetus has inherited the normal gene. Here the fetus is at low risk, because the only way it could have inherited the mutant gene is if a chromosome breakage and exchange event has occurred between the linked marker and the gene.

Genes Do Not Function in Isolation; Environment Counts

Legendary football coach Vince Lombardi once said, "Winning isn't everything, it's the only thing." When it comes to our body's health, genetics is certainly neither everything, nor is it the "only thing." Despite the substantial influence that genes have on bodily activities, we must keep in mind that genes, while important, are not the only determining factors. The effects that genes have on our health are greatly influenced by the environment in which they function. This environment can be as limited as the internal conditions of a cell, as temporary as the intra-uterine world of the developing fetus, or as enormous as the vast array of external physical, chemical, and cultural factors that constitute the larger world in which we live. Sometimes the environment can have a small impact, mildly altering the way a gene works or the effect that its presence ultimately has on the individual. At other times, the environmental influences can be substantial and decisive, completely camouflaging the presence of some genes or markedly intensifying the action of others.

Even if we know that a certain mutant gene is present, it may not be possible to predict how that gene will finally be expressed and what the outcome on health will be, either at the time of birth or later on as the individual develops and matures. Different mutations in the same gene can have different effects on health—from being unnoticeable to causing severe problems. Even the *same* mutation can affect different people differently. For instance, a tiny change in one of the genes responsible for making a part of the hemoglobin molecule found in our red blood cells may, in one person, result in a severe life-threatening form of sickle-cell anemia. Someone else, with exactly the same genetic mutation, may have a very mild case. As another example, the presence of a particular set of genes may predispose some individuals in a family to cancer or heart disease that will develop later in their lives. But other family members with the same genetic makeup may well be spared.

Despite our increased understanding of human genes and the growing constellation of genetic tests, the complex collaboration between the contribution of the genes and the contribution of the environment remains a mystery.

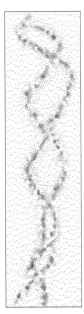

Chapter Three

Finding Out about Genetic Tests

N early every day, it seems, we hear of dramatic new discoveries from the field of genetics. A newspaper article announces that a gene connected with a serious health problem has been identified. Or a report describes a new genetic test that can tell if a particular gene is flawed or not. Or a TV news feature speculates that new ways to correct defects in DNA might be the ultimate treatment for genetic illness. From all the visibility that this field has achieved, it would seem a simple matter to locate the medical professionals who have expertise in matters of genetics. It would appear to be relatively straightforward to get explanations and help in answering at least some of the questions that the families we met in Chapter One are asking.

All too often the reality is quite different. Finding genetic information in the medical community is frequently frustrating and difficult. This is especially the case when a genetic disorder is first diagnosed, or when the possibility suddenly arises that a particular individual might have some sort of flawed gene. Granted, many people do succeed in getting to the appropriate specialists in genetic medicine. However, many others never do make their way through the health-care system to gain the information they would like to have. And many more acquire their basic knowledge indirectly, from second- or third-hand sources, especially from others in their own family. They rely on genetic information that has been gathered at some point by a family member and which has been passed along from person to person through the family. This informal network, of information sharing and exchange among family members, I call a "genetic grapevine." It is this genetic grapevine that consumers often use to estimate what their own genetic risks might be, and to guide their own choices about having genetic tests.

In this chapter we will focus on the places *within* the health-care community where consumers can go for genetic information, and what they can expect when they get there. Suggestions provided by many consumers who have taken part in what is generally called "genetic counseling" will highlight what can be done to gain the most benefit from that experience. We will see how misunderstandings arise. Later on, in Chapter Eight, we will see what other ways there are to obtain accurate and up-to-date information about genetic tools, tests, and treatments—ways that supplement standard medical practice and which can be useful to those who count on the genetic grapevine to keep themselves informed.

Sources of Genetic Information in the Medical Community

As with any problem that affects our health, it is natural to turn to medical professionals. Whether one has allergies or heart problems or back pain, there is usually a family doctor or a medical specialist to check out what is happening, order tests, interpret the results, and recommend courses of treatment. But where does one go for a problem when there are genes involved? Where in the health-care system can the genetic gurus be found?

Genetic specialists can be found in special units or divisions of many hospitals and medical centers, as well as in private centers. These units may be variously named: medical genetics, human genetics, pediatric genetics, clinical genetics, and genetic counseling. Sometimes, genetic specialists are based in clinics that deal with a specific type of condition such as hemophilia or neuromuscular disorders or breast cancer.

At any of these units there may be physicians, researchers, counselors, social workers, and nurses, all of whom have special training in genetics. Usually working in a group and functioning as a team, genetic professionals carry out a range of activities. To simplify matters, the term "genetic counseling" will be used to describe the kinds of services that these professionals provide.

What genetic professionals will offer clients will differ, depending on the individual situation of each client. This may include:

- making an assessment of what the family's health problems are, and explaining the hereditary basis of those problems;
- collecting the data that could help establish whether the client (as well as other present or future family members) is at risk for developing a genetic disorder, and estimating what the risk might be;
- explaining the types of testing and treatment that are available and assisting the client in pursuing genetic testing or other options if they are chosen;
- providing support to people experiencing the practical problems and emotional distress that a genetic disorder may bring on.

Finding out where these genetic services are is not an easy matter. It is not as simple as turning to the Yellow Pages of the local phone book. Genetic services, embedded as they are within the confines of other medical specialties, can be hard to track down. Usually the family physician or other primary-care provider or specialist makes the referral.

Many questions about the possibility of inherited illness naturally come up during pregnancy. The obstetrician has become one of the main figures in the medical system who identifies those who have a genetic disorder, or who may be at risk for one, and who puts these clients in contact with a genetic counseling program. For example, pregnant women over age thirty-five are offered genetic counseling and testing because of their increased risk of having a child with abnormalities in chromosome number. Prospective parents belonging to a group with a higher risk of being carriers of a gene for a particular disorder—such as sickle-cell anemia in African American individuals, thalassemia (a group of hereditary anemias) in people from Mediterranean countries, or Tay-Sachs disease in Ashkenazic Jewish individuals— are also offered genetic tests during pregnancy.

Provision of such access to genetic information and testing for pregnant women has rapidly been incorporated into prenatal care—so rapidly in fact, that some genetic tests may come to be regarded as routine. Feminist scholars and others have voiced serious concerns about what they see as a medical assembly line in which genetic testing to establish the chromosome number of the fetus and to determine the possible carrier status of the parents will be viewed as an automatic part of prenatal care. They fear that women will be given little or no say about whether they really want to have these tests.

The situation may be quite different when a genetic disorder suddenly bursts on the scene, as it has for the Stone, MacFarlane, and Tate families. Here the road to genetic counseling services is uncertain. Many people find themselves stranded, left without any road map that could guide them to the genetic information they wish to have. The circumstances under which a genetic disorder is diagnosed or a potential problem surfaces are at the heart of the difference.

Coming abruptly, as it usually does, the awareness of a genetic problem can evoke strong and painful responses. Those who have experienced this use such phrases as "traumatic," "shocking," "devastating," "a kick in the head," "a bolt from the blue," to try to describe how they felt. One couple said they were a "total wreck." Men who had never before allowed themselves to cry gave in to tears.

It is a time of great stress for the doctor as well. There are so many matters that demand immediate attention, from caring for a patient with urgent health problems, to dealing with the feelings of loss, desperation, and grief. At such moments, a discussion about the hereditary aspects of the health problem may not even come up. If it occurs at all, it tends to be perfunctory. The possibility of a referral elsewhere for genetic counseling may be shunted into the background and, ultimately, forgotten.

Then too, the person making the diagnosis—a family doctor, a pediatrician, a neurologist, or any one of a variety of other specialists—may not know the details of the inheritance patterns or be current on the latest findings in genetic research. That this should be the case is unfortunate but not surprising. Until recently, genetics has not been prominently featured in medical training. Most of the single-gene disorders are rare and are seldom, if ever, seen by most health-care specialists. The genetic contribution to the more common health problems that physicians are likely to be quite familiar with is complicated. Genetic research is proceeding at a feverish pace, with new DNA tests appearing continually. It requires a considerable investment of time for medical professionals to keep current with genetic advances, along with everything else that bids for their attention.

Then, too, not everyone is sitting in a doctor's office when he or she first hears about genetic illness or the risk of such illness. Many people get this news from another family member. Set in motion by those who first get the diagnosis, word of a genetic problem can cascade through families, spreading over long distances and across generations. In person, by phone, through Christmas letters, by every mode of communication that is used to stay in touch, relatives obtain information and, in turn, may pass it along to others. The amount of genetic information that percolates through the family network will depend on how much was given at the start of the chain. All too often, it will be minimal. Even worse, by the time the information has passed through many stages of repetition, it may be altered and unreliable.

Despite all the different obstacles that can get in the way, consumers who seek genetic information can be successful in finding a genetic counseling center. The first, and most obvious, step is to ask for a referral from a primary-care physician or from the physician who specializes in the disorder of concern. Another step that consumers can take is to contact the National Society of Genetic Counselors or the Council of Regional Networks for Genetic Services. (See Section I of the Appendix for address and telephone information.) Either of these organizations can direct consumers to genetic counseling centers in their region. State health departments, located in the state capital, are another way of finding out where genetic counseling activities are taking place. Ask for the office of the genetic services director or coordinator.

Categories of Genetic Tests, and Their Uses

Genetic tests—the original forms as well as the new DNA tests—may be conducted at different times in a life cycle, depending on the type of information being sought.

Prenatal tests are tests performed on the genetic material of fetal or placental cells collected during the early stages of pregnancy, using procedures such as amniocentesis or chorionic villus sampling (discussed in Chapter Two). Prenatal tests are done to find out whether the child will have a particular genetic disorder at birth or will develop it at some point afterward. For example, there is a DNA linkage test that Andrew and Donna Stone could use to learn the likelihood that their next child will be born having inherited two recessive genes, one from each of them. This double-recessive scenario will lead to spinal muscular atrophy, the same condition that affected their first child.

Carrier tests done on blood samples (or on other easily obtained tissue samples, such as cells gently scraped off the mouth lining) are used to identify those individuals who possess a single copy of a mutant gene. This type of test is performed when there is reason to believe, based on family history or the higher frequency of a mutation in a population group, that an individual could have a single copy of a gene for a disorder. Such individuals (called carriers), while perfectly healthy themselves, could pass that gene on to children where its effects may show up. Jackie MacFarlane and her sisters could opt for such a test to find out if they are carriers of the gene located on the X chromosome that is associated with Duchenne muscular dystrophy. Female carriers of the gene are at risk for having sons with that disorder. (As discussed in Chapter Two, this occurs because males have only one X chromosome and they get that chromosome from their mother. Females are protected by the genes contained on their second X chromosome.)

Presymptomatic tests are yet another category of genetic test. Such tests are used when a currently healthy person wants to know if a flawed gene is present, a gene whose effects usually do not appear until later on in life. This person already knows a risk exists because a relative actually has the disorder. The test permits that individual to learn whether he or she will develop the disorder, before any symptoms appear. For some late-onset disorders, a careful physical examination with standard diagnostic procedures may be sufficient to reveal the earliest stages. Presymptomatic testing can be useful when early signs are absent or undetectable. Huntington disease, a disorder which usually begins to reveal itself in the fourth or fifth decade of life, is the classic example in this category.

Susceptibility tests are used to determine if a gene or genes are present that may predispose a person to developing a health problem later on in life. This newest category of genetic test is designed to look for genes associated with illnesses as diverse as some types of cancer, heart disease, diabetes, and possibly Alzheimer's disease or bipolar disorder. A susceptibility test can only tell (from the genes that are present) whether it is more likely or less likely that the disorder will occur. If the test detects the presence of such predisposing genes, this indicates a higher-than-average probability that the disorder will develop (perhaps decades down the road)—but there is no certainty that it will develop. If the test shows the absence of those genes, then the person has an average chance of developing the disorder. In this case, of course, there is still no guarantee that it will not occur.

There are important complications. One is the fact that, for each disorder, there are often several different predisposing genes. Some of these have not yet been identified, so they cannot be tested for. In addition, it is known that all of these illnesses involve a host of environmental factors. Factors such as diet, amount of exercise, and exposure to certain types of pollutants or disease germs can contribute to the onset of such disorders. There are also environmental factors that are not yet understood. Sophie Baldwin might consider being tested for genes that, if present, predispose her to breast cancer.

Oftentimes both presymptomatic and susceptibility tests are referred to as "predictive tests." But it is important to realize that the two categories of tests provide different types of prediction. A presymptomatic test checks for a mutant gene *which must be present* for the disorder to occur. The disorder will not appear unless the damaged gene or genes are present. A susceptibility test checks for a gene whose presence can increase the chances of developing a disorder. The disorder may not develop even if the damaged gene is present, and it may develop even if the damaged gene is absent. In order to avoid confusing one genetic situation with the other, I will not use the term "predictive test" elsewhere in this book.

What the Genetic Counseling Team Can and Cannot Do

A visit to a genetic counseling service can provide information and understanding about the nature of the disorder. It can also provide access to genetic testing, if that is desired. Other options, including family planning alternatives, may be offered. This is not counseling in the traditional sense, where there is usually an ongoing relationship between the counselor and the client. For the most part, genetic counseling is a short-term arrangement which can be renewed from time to time when new questions, new family realities, or test options arise.

As part of genetic counseling, medical geneticists will work to confirm a diagnosis, providing a name and a set of known features to the condition in question. They may conclude that the condition is not genetic but arises from other causes such as infection, inadequate oxygen at birth, nutritional deficiencies, or other, as yet unidentified, external factors. Where the diagnosis is definite and genetic in origin, then genetic counseling provides the means for educating the client and exploring the available choices. Opportunities for genetic testing are a major topic of discussion. Through genetic counseling, one can learn the details of how a particular genetic test is carried out and what it determines. This information would include the accuracy and limitations of the test, the costs and time required, and the options that are available once the results are obtained. For some disorders, such as Huntington disease, there is a defined set of procedures (or protocol) that is followed and this will need to be explained. With such testing, many steps are built in to allow each person to think through the choice carefully and to permit adequate follow-up once the results are in.

What consumers can *not* expect from genetic counseling is that they will be told what course of action to take. Genetic specialists, no matter what form of training they have had, hold firmly to a professional code that calls for complete neutrality in their work. This neutral, or as they call it "nondirective," approach is meant to keep the decision making in the control of the clients. Whether it is really possible for the genetic specialist to be completely nondirective, to give no hint at all of his or her own personal feelings, is, of course, doubtful. Still, genetic counselors are committed to the view that they must avoid imposing their own beliefs and choices on anyone else. So it is the consumer who is the ultimate decision maker in matters of genetic testing.

Nor will the genetic counseling team actively search out other family members and urge them to come in to have their own genetic risk determined. And they will not contact relatives of a client and persuade them to provide blood samples so that linkage testing can be carried out. For ethical and practical reasons, the genetic professionals will not and cannot take on these obligations. It is the consumers themselves who are the first line of contact with their own families. They must be the ones to bring genetic issues to the attention of other family members and to let them know that genetic counseling services are available. They are the ones who must explain to family members why their blood samples are a necessary part of someone else's test. As we shall see in Chapter Four, this expectation that the consumer be the one to reach out to other relatives can complicate some forms of genetic testing, and, in fact, can be a barrier to it.

What Consumers Can and Cannot Do

More than to any other type of medical interaction, the consumer brings to the genetic counseling process an expertise that is crucial. The consumer is not just an individual with questions and problems that someone with specialized training can help resolve. He or she is part of a family unit, and in this way is connected to others who share some of the same genetic endowment. He or she may be concerned about what this genetic connection may mean for the health of family members and for the well-being of those not yet born. The consumer's in-depth knowledge of this family tree and the relationships within it is of vital importance. In addition, any person who has cared for children or parents with a disorder has a wealth of hard-won practical experience which rivals the textbook knowledge that a medical expert can contribute.

To make the best use of the time and to get the most out of a genetic counseling session, consumers should be prepared to provide a key item, *an accurate and complete family history.* For any genetic assessment to be carried out, it is necessary to find out who the members are in the nuclear family and in the extended family and exactly how they are related. Further, it is important to know what health problems they have or, if they have died, what they did have. The genetic specialists use the family history, which they organize into a diagram, as the basis for identifying what the genetic problems may be and for providing estimates of risk.

Often, putting a family history or family tree together is just a matter of remembering and writing down the information. In some families, there may be an older aunt, uncle, or grandparent who can shed light on the family's past history. A relative with an interest in genealogy may have already gathered and recorded much of this material. But, sometimes, even within small families, this information can be hard to come by. Facts about earlier generations may have been lost over time. Current generations may be hard to describe because of geographical distance, divorce, death, or disagreements, circumstances that can isolate family members from one another. Some relatives may not understand why details about their siblings or children are being sought. They may get angry and object to having anyone poke into their private lives. People may not reveal that there had been children who had been put up for adoption, pregnancies that were terminated, or liaisons that produced children outside of marriage.

Genetic counseling is also dependent on having an accurate diagnosis and an understanding of the family health history. Tracking the family's health history may be another problem. In the past, many disorders were simply never spoken of, especially if they caused early or untimely death. Parents, diagnosed with a genetic illness, may find it too painful to share that fact with their children. Until recently, even a common illness like cancer has been a taboo subject in many families.

Further complications arise when the same disorder has been known by different names over the years, making it difficult for a person to track a disorder over generations. For example, the term "night-blindness" is no longer used; "retinitis pigmentosa" is now the preferred term. "Neurofibromatosis type 1" is the preferred designation for what previously was called von Recklinghausen disease. The name "spinal muscular atrophy" is now used for a set of closely related disorders that once carried names like Werdnig-Hoffman disease and Kugelberg-Welander syndrome. Fragile-X syndrome, a recently defined condition, was designated in the past with broadly descriptive terms such as "minimal brain damage" and "mental retardation."

Sometimes a family invents a special name for a health problem. These special names make identifying family health problems even more confusing. Nicknames for illnesses abound because they are simpler to say than the official medical term and sound less frightening. By giving a disorder a familiar label, family members are able to more comfortably weave the disorder into their daily lives. For instance, one family uses "the old man's complaint" when they talk about Huntington disease. Another prefers "stiff-foot disease" to Charcot-Marie-Tooth disease, or "the eye problem" to retinitis pigmentosa. All the variations in terminology can make it appear that there are different disorders in different parts of the family. In some cases, this masquerade of names can disguise the fact that a single disorder is involved, and that it may be genetic in origin. In order to establish the correct diagnosis (or, failing that, to gain an accurate description of the family health problems), genetic specialists may request permission to search medical records if such records are still available. They may need to arrange physical examinations and diagnostic tests on family members.

An accurate picture of the family is more than just a valuable aid to genetic specialists. It is also an essential tool for setting up DNA tests and interpreting the results of these tests. Mistakes in the way family relationships or health problems are described can have serious consequences. A low-risk result may be given to someone who is actually at high risk, or vice versa. In prenatal testing, erroneous conclusions about the genetic makeup of the fetus may be drawn. Consumers should be aware that, even with their best efforts to gather accurate family histories, mistakes can be made in the diagnosis of the illness or in the drawing of the family tree. Both types of mistakes are the source of potential error in genetic testing.

Often, errors in test results arise when a man who is shown on the family history diagram as the father of a child is not, in fact, the biological father. This is a situation commonly called "nonpaternity" or, more accurately, "wrong paternity." Linkage testing is especially vulnerable to errors stemming from wrong paternity, since an incorrect family tree can confuse the identification of the markers that are traveling with the target gene. Identifying the wrong man as the biological father can result in the wrong marker being used as the DNA signal followed in linkage testing. This yields linkage test results that are completely invalid. Consumers aware of the possibility of wrong paternity should share this fact, in confidence, with a member of the counseling team. Wrong paternity or misrepresentation occurring elsewhere in the family tree will be hard to guard against. Children may not have any inkling that the man they know as their father is not really their biological father, or that one of their cousins was the child of an extramarital affair.

In general, the consumer will have to abide by the policies adopted by the genetic counseling service—policies that provide a framework for the way different types of testing will be carried out. These policies, or protocols, are plans describing how counseling and testing for a particular disorder should be carried out. A protocol details all the steps that must be taken and the minimum time that has to be set aside for each step. It may impose restrictions on testing of fetuses or children. A protocol is generally the result of prior research studies and is intended to provide the most benefit with the least harm for clients. Protocols for Huntington disease were among the first developed. Many places have established their own protocols for other disorders as well. Policies do evolve and change. Genetic professionals are also sensitive to the need to modify a protocol where special circumstances prevail, and will do so if possible. Typically, however, consumers may not omit steps or speed up the pace of the genetic counseling and of any testing that they select.

In some cases, DNA samples may be sent to a research laboratory if there happens to be a laboratory studying the genetic basis for a particular disorder. Because a research laboratory is not run as a business and is not set up to provide testing services in the routine way a commercial laboratory does, the turnaround time to get information back may be slow. Much will depend on the laboratory's workload and its ability to fit the testing of a few samples in with all its other research functions. If samples are intended solely for study in a research program, they may be stored for long periods of time until the investigators are ready to begin their experimental studies. Consumers who decide to donate samples for future research purposes should find out whether the laboratory is planning to share with them what they discover about their genes whenever their sample is eventually studied. A fuller discussion on research activities and how consumers can help further such investigations will be found in Chapter Seven.

Getting the Most from Genetic Counseling

Going for genetic counseling can be like traveling to another land. The location may be an unfamiliar and distant place. The people working there will be strangers to the consumer. And the language they speak may contain so many medical and genetic terms that it sounds like a foreign language. Consumers who have had genetic counseling have offered suggestions—some travel tips, so to speak—for feeling more comfortable and for making the visit the most useful and relevant to their needs.

Their suggestions start with the making of the appointment itself. It is wise, according to consumers who are veterans of genetic counseling, to *choose the time carefully*. The ideal time is when the person or the parents will be in a frame of mind that will allow them to learn the most and benefit most fully from genetic counseling. Genetic educators call this the "teachable moment." There are many such moments and they occur at different times for different people. Those who live at a distance from the genetic counseling service may not have much choice; their meeting with the counselors may be decided by when they can make the trip.

Of those who can pick the time more easily, a few will want to know as much as they can right away. Others will want to wait. For one couple, it was important that they have genetic counseling within a few days of learning that their son had spinal muscular atrophy. Their ability to cope with their son's condition depended on having as full a sense of the genetic story as possible. They were relieved to learn that this condition came from an unlucky throw of the genetic dice and that they hadn't done anything themselves to cause it. It made dealing with their feelings of loss, anger, grief, and mourning much easier. It also allowed them to begin to plan for the future.

Others have found that the first few weeks, even months, after getting their child's diagnosis are so difficult, mentally and physically, that they are overwhelmed, left completely drained, or "emotionally hung over," as one woman called it. It takes time to accept the reality that your child has a serious condition. People who have had counseling during this period may be too tired and too distracted to get much out of it. Many genetic counselors believe that crisis situations take such a toll that they disempower people. If this is the case, consumers should postpone genetic counseling until things have settled down. Consumers can still use this interval to slowly gather the family information that will be so important to the genetic counseling they eventually receive.

By medical standards, a genetic counseling appointment can be lengthy, lasting about an hour in many cases. It needs to be this long because a great deal of territory has to be covered. There are many studies which show how hard it is for consumers to understand and retain the information they were given when they had genetic counseling. No wonder! Most likely during that session many genetic concepts and terms, mostly unfamiliar, were used and defined. If the relevant tests exist, this fact and some of the strengths and shortcomings of the tests probably had to be explained as well. A variety of medical options and alternatives, including reproductive ones, may have been discussed.

Consumers have offered several strategies to help reduce the inevitable gaps in understanding that occur when this mass of material is presented.

Make a record of what is being said. This can be as simple as taking along a pen and paper to write key items down. It can mean using a tape recorder so that parts of the session can be reviewed afterward.

Try to bring someone, a trusted relative or friend, who can listen along with you. Having more listeners helps increase comprehension. What one person does not catch, another might. One couple brought along several friends and relatives in order to have "as many ears as possible." Later, when they talked together about what they heard, they realized that each one had missed a lot. However, when the information was shared, a more complete and accurate picture emerged that enhanced their overall understanding.

Reduce distractions. Don't bring along children or anyone whose presence may increase anxiety or divert attention away from the issues being discussed. One couple realized it had been a mistake to bring their two young children along to the genetic counseling session. The constant interruptions from the corner of the office where they were playing made it hard for the parents to focus on what the genetic counselor was saying.

Ask that statistical or numerical information be explained in different ways. Part of what consumers expect from genetic counseling is that they will get an explanation, in understandable terms, of genetic and medical matters that are of concern to them. This is also the goal of the genetic professionals at that session. Therefore, it is important that consumers clearly indicate when they do not understand something. Genetic professionals want to get this type of feedback. A 25 percent chance of having an affected child at each pregnancy means there is a 75 percent chance (or three chances out of four) that the child will *not* be affected. A DNA test result that is 97 percent accurate means that for three people in one hundred, the test result will be incorrect. To fathom what the numbers mean, it helps to hear them expressed in different ways.

Clarify the meaning of the words that are used. Because of the many scientific terms, it is not surprising that the language of genetics can be especially hard to understand. What adds an extra layer of confusion is that seemingly familiar words can mean something very unfamiliar and different when used by genetic specialists. It is always a good idea to ask for clarification of how words are being used.

Here are some examples to show how ordinary English words can be misunderstood. Medical people use the word "positive" (as in, "your test results are positive") to mean that the test has revealed a problem or a malfunction. In genetic testing, a positive result means that a malfunctioning gene or genes are present. This is very different from general usage, in which the word "positive" usually connotes something desirable (as in, "She has a really positive outlook on life") or certain ("I'm positive he will be there"). In a genetic setting, this drastic difference in meaning has led to confusion. One woman was convinced, based on getting a positive result for the presence of the gene for Huntington disease, that the report was good and that she had been spared any further concern. It was her understanding that any bad news would be reflected in a "negative" result. Another person thought that his positive result only meant that the doctors would know for sure whether he had the gene or not.

Other common words have been the source of confusion. Told that his was an "isolated case," one man with neurofibromatosis assumed that the disorder, caused when a single dominant gene is present, was a single occurrence that would stay with him but would not go on to his children. Even though he is the first member of his family to have the disorder (most likely because a new mutation occurred), there is a 50 percent chance at each pregnancy that the mutated gene will be passed to a child who will then show signs of the disorder. Another family concluded erroneously that "dominant" meant that something was more frequent—that "dominated" in a group of children. So they believed that spinal muscular atrophy must be dominant because, in their own family, two of their three children had the disorder. Since spinal muscular atrophy occurs when two recessive mutant genes come together, their real risk of having an affected child at the next pregnancy is 25 percent, not 50 percent, as it would be for a disorder brought on by a dominant gene.

Request that you be given a written summary and other materials to review later. It is essential to have information that can be used as a source of reference after the genetic counseling session is over. This can be in the form of a letter summarizing what was discussed and containing the especially important items of information. Brochures about the disorder or material describing genetic tests may also be available, along with pamphlets provided by support groups for people facing similar concerns.

Find out who in the group should be contacted if you want more information or if DNA testing is going to be done. The need to communicate with genetic specialists may be ongoing. Questions will certainly surface after the genetic counseling session. Other family members, considering whether to have testing, may wish to consult with a genetic specialist as they sort out their thoughts. It is a good idea to know the most efficient and direct way to get in touch.

Trends in Genetic Testing

Genetic counseling has been the traditional gateway to genetic testing. Not only is the counseling service the source of information about what genetic tests are available; currently it is also the base of operations that enables the tests to be carried out. The genetic counseling group arranges for the collection and sending of samples, and, after test results are received, it interprets them and provides any follow-up that is needed.

This situation is changing. As more and more doctors become part of managed health-care arrangements, they will be facing substantial pressures from within their health-care organizations to control costs. Such financial constraints may make the primary-care doctor reluctant to authorize a referral to any specialists, including genetic specialists. There is already a noticeable tendency among obstetricians and doctors in other medical specialties not to refer their clients to genetic counseling services but to provide genetic information themselves and handle all the arrangements for carrying out any genetic tests. At the same time there are also growing efforts by commercial laboratories to market genetic tests to doctors, especially tests for susceptibility to common health problems.

All of these trends make it likely that, in the future, more DNA testing will be handled by primary-care physicians and by doctors practicing in neurology, internal medicine, oncology, and other specialties. Genetic counseling units may be bypassed in the process. If these circumstances arise, consumers should request that their health-care provider give them detailed genetic information about the disorder, spell out the available options for testing, and discuss what kind of information the test can and cannot provide. The strategies described above for getting the most out of a meeting with professionals in a genetic counseling center can be implemented in other health-care settings as well.

Regardless of where the information is given and how all the details are handled, the ultimate decision about having a genetic test should remain where it has always been—with the consumer. In the next chapter, we examine how consumers make such decisions.

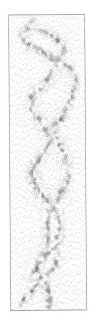

Chapter Four

Making Decisions about Genetic Testing

Intense research activity in scientific laboratories has led to the development of a new type of medical measuring stick: the DNA test. In such a test, the genetic material is examined to gain information about the condition of a particular gene, just as a stethoscope is used to check the condition of the heart and lungs in the doctor's office. There are two general types of DNA tests, as I have discussed in Chapter Two. A *direct test* can be done when an inherited disorder is connected with known alterations in a gene. Here the test is precise enough to indicate the presence or absence of specific flaws in the gene. Direct tests are possible for many disorders including Huntington disease, cystic fibrosis, and sickle-cell anemia. A *linkage test* can be done when the alterations in the gene (and when even the gene itself) are not known. Here the test can still provide clues or predictions about the nature of the genes that are present. Linkage tests are used for disorders such as neurofibromatosis, Duchenne muscular dystrophy, and spinal muscular atrophy.

Just because a genetic test becomes available does *not* mean that everyone takes the next step and has the test. Some do. Some make the opposite choice and decide against it. Still others postpone the decision until a later time. In this chapter we look at the factors that affect an individual's decision to undergo or forgo genetic testing. The focus here will be on genetic testing for the so-called single-gene disorders, in which one or both copies of a given gene can trigger changes that hamper health. In Chapter Five disorders such as cancer and heart disease will be discussed. In these complex disorders, genes at different places on the chromosomes combine with environmental factors to initiate the disease.

There are a number of published studies describing decisions consumers have made about genetic tests in use since the late 1960s. Such "classic" tests include the microscope-based tests, which look at the chromosome number and structure, as well as biochemical analyses which figure out genetic makeup by looking at the protein products produced by genes. However, the character of DNA testing is very different from these earlier forms. DNA tests have made it possible to explore medical areas that earlier genetic tests could not. Thus experience with the earlier tests cannot be used as the sole guide for decisions about the new DNA tests.

Huntington disease is one of the disorders for which DNA tests were first developed. Affecting about thirty thousand people in the United States, Huntington disease occurs when a single copy of a mutant gene brings about the gradual loss of a cluster of cells in a portion of the brain known as the basal ganglia, which controls involuntary muscle movement. As the number of these cells decreases, the ceaseless muscle movements typical of the disorder begin. The involuntary muscle movements and other signs of mental deterioration are not noticeable until midlife, usually long after a person with the gene has had children. There is a 50 percent chance that each child could receive the Huntington disease gene from an affected parent.

Though rare, Huntington disease was brought to prominence when Woody Guthrie, a leading folk singer and song writer, died from it. His wife, Marjorie, later joined by others, spearheaded drives to raise interest in understanding and curing this disease and to obtain funds that would support research. The research activities were aided in great part by people living in several communities near Lake Maracaibo in Venezuela, where the incidence of Huntington disease was high. The disease first appeared in that region at some point in the distant past. Because of the interconnections among the communities, high birth rates, and the stability of the population, the people living there became, over time, an enormous extended family composed of some thirteen thousand members. Studies begun in the early 1980s to find the disease gene were greatly aided by carefully figuring out the relationships of the people in these communities to each other and by collecting hundreds of blood samples from affected and unaffected family members. With these blood samples, plus some pure luck in selecting DNA markers that just happened to be located near the target gene, it became possible by the mid-1980s to do DNA linkage testing for the Huntington disease gene.

Since then, intense interest in Huntington disease testing has made it into a model for all types of DNA testing procedures and policies. The experience with testing for Huntington disease has contributed a lot to our understanding of the factors that need to be taken into account when considering genetic testing. However, the pattern of late onset and the nature of the symptoms of Huntington disease make this disorder a rather special case. Thus, it cannot be used as a model for DNA testing in general. Nor can it represent the needs and issues relevant to testing for other types of genetic disorders.

Perhaps the most valuable way to gain deeper insight into the factors that must be considered when contemplating DNA testing is to listen to the voices of those who find themselves on the genetic testing frontier. Most notable among these are the individuals (like the Stones, MacFarlanes, Tates, and Baldwins) who are faced with the necessity to consider such testing for themselves or loved ones. As we have before, we will use the inadequate term "consumers" to describe all such candidates for testing. Also involved are the professional geneticists and genetic counselors with whom consumers interact. Drawing on the real-world experience of those who have been directly concerned with a wide variety of genetic disorders, and who have themselves been candidates for DNA testing, we can tap into a rich resource of information and insight.

I arranged over eighty interviews with individuals who shared with me their experience about DNA testing. They are a diverse group of people living in different geographic areas; from different ethnic, religious, and racial groups; and at different places on educational and income ladders. Their accounts provided a rich source of information about people's interactions with this new technology. Their stories include experiences with tests for recessive, X-linked, and dominantly inherited conditions. Among these are spinal muscular atrophy, Duchenne muscular dystrophy, Coffin-Lowry syndrome, cystic fibrosis, neurofibromatosis, and retinitis pigmentosa. Some had undergone genetic testing; others decided not to. These were *not* the unusual or sensational stories—the thorny, complicated, perplexing situations that form the grist for ethics debates or courtroom confrontations or TV specials. These were the more usual stories. They depicted typical genetic-testing situations. Each story of course was different, reflecting the unique features and circumstances that characterize each and every human situation. And yet, by revealing the fundamental similarities that underlie genetic decision making, each contributed to providing a picture of genetic testing both in broad outline and in the fine detail. The observations of professional geneticists in research laboratories, genetic counseling clinics, and other health-care settings supplement and complement the profound experiences of the consumers.

From these accounts, four general factors emerge as central in decisions regarding DNA testing:

- the specific characteristics of the *disorder* for which testing is being offered, as well as the nature of current treatments and the prospects for better therapeutic interventions;
- the requirements of the *test* itself, including such aspects as how many other family members need to be involved, how long it takes before results are obtained, how accurate the results are, and how much the testing process costs;
- the age of the individual and his or her circumstances at the *time* that testing is being considered;
- the new *options* or opportunities that might be opened up as a result of obtaining the test results and, conversely, the options or opportunities that would be closed off.

Let's now look more closely at each of these four factors.

The Disorder

One key component in any decision about undergoing genetic testing is the nature and severity of the disorder itself. Questions about neurofibromatosis that Phyllis Tate, for example, will ask herself include the following. At what age do the symptoms start to show up? What health problems appear? Is the condition stable or does it get worse over time? What is the degree of disability or discomfort that occurs? And will it be possible for a person with it to still have children?

Sometimes these questions can be directly answered. Someone who already has a disorder knows the answers firsthand. This firsthand knowledge is a powerful tool in assessing the desirability of genetic testing for one's own children or potential children. Someone who has observed the disorder in relatives can also know a good deal about it. With dominant or late-onset disorders, older members of the family may be affected. With recessive disorders, there may be a previously affected baby, child, or sibling. When X-linked genes are involved, there may be male relatives—brothers, uncles, or cousins—with the genetic illness.

Personal experience does have its limitations. One's own experience can be inadequate for judging a progressive disorder; later, and perhaps more severe, stages have not yet been seen. Observations based on older relatives can be misleading if available therapies have improved over time. Even when personal knowledge is quite recent, the presence of other genes or additional environmental factors may produce wide variation in symptoms. Even siblings with the same disorder can differ markedly in the way that the disorder develops. One mother was struck by dramatic differences in the manner that neurofibromatosis progressed in her two children; the older child had much milder symptoms than the younger.

When there is no direct experience to call on, consumers have sought to obtain information about the disorder in a variety of ways. They have turned to members of the medical community, to national organizations and local support groups concerned with the disorder, to the popular press, and even to the medical literature itself. Further details on the types of resources available and ways of gaining access to them can be found in Chapter Eight and the Appendix.

In addition to questions about the nature and severity of the disorder, there are important questions about the range of therapies and services that can be used to deal with it. Are scientists close to a cure? If not, are there effective medical treatments available? Would the caregiver be sufficiently adept at, or comfortable with, the day-to-day responsibilities of looking after someone affected with the disorder? Are treatments generally available nearby, or would it be necessary to travel to medical centers located elsewhere in the country? Is the price affordable? What other kinds of services—educational, occupational, social—can be called upon to assist an affected individual? Might improvements in treatments and services be reasonably expected to occur?

The ease and effectiveness of the available treatments are important to consumers. Genetic counselors report many situations in which individuals have preferred to rely on treatment rather than utilize genetic tests. For example, few families choose to be tested for the gene related to the mild-to-moderate forms of hemophilia, although this test would help identify female carriers and affected male fetuses. The reason for this choice is the availability of effective treatments for the blood clotting problem of mild-to-moderate hemophilia. Similarly, many of those at risk for the adult-onset form of polycystic kidney disease decline presymptomatic testing. For them, it is preferable to rely on tests for kidney structure and function that indicate that there will be kidney problems, and then to use current treatments, including kidney transplantation, when they are needed. By contrast, when Duchenne muscular dystrophy is the issue, the *absence* of effective treatment is often cited by parents as the main reason for seeking carrier testing and prenatal testing.

The Test

At some point in our lives, most of us have had occasion to undergo some form of medical testing. Usually, no matter how sick we may have felt, the testing itself was a fairly simple matter. Perhaps it was a cotton swab grazing our throat to see if we had a strep infection, or a urine sample collected to check for infection, or a blood sample drawn to test for substances that could identify how one or the other of our internal organs was faring. Whatever form the testing took, the necessary sample came from our own body alone. And the results, obtained within hours or at the most a few days, usually gave a clear indication about what was or wasn't bothering us. Though we rarely thought about it, we realized that there is always a very small chance of getting a wrong test result through some kind of error such as a sample mix-up or a shortcoming in the laboratory procedures.

On the surface, DNA tests appear to be no different. The consumer provides blood or some other type of tissue sample from which the genetic material is extracted for subsequent examination. The end result is an answer about the status of a particular gene. However, DNA tests have some facets that should be kept in mind. Some DNA tests require the consumer to make additional decisions and take other actions before the actual testing can begin. There can be still further complications when it comes to interpreting the results. Consumers have found that these additional features introduce elements that play a central part in their decision about whether or not to have DNA testing, especially for the linkage type of DNA testing.

Direct DNA Tests

For an increasing number of single-gene disorders, direct DNA testing is not only feasible, it is the testing method of choice. The person seeking the genetic information need only provide a blood or tissue sample and then wait for a relatively brief time for the results. Although in most ways direct testing differs little from other standard kinds of diagnostic tests, the results can be less conclusive than they may first appear. For direct DNA test results to be interpreted accurately, it is necessary to know what the precise mutation is. For some disorders, such as sickle-cell anemia, there is only one mutation, so those with the sickle-cell gene are easily identified by the presence of that characteristic mutation in their DNA. For most other disorders, however, there are usually other mutations in a gene that interfere with its function.

For the direct test to be useful, it must be able to detect the *specific* mutation that appears in the consumer's family. As indicated earlier, sometimes mutations are family specific. Thus it is important to determine what that mutation is by examining the DNA from an affected person—that is, from the person in the family who already has the disorder. Once testing of the DNA has been done for the affected person, information about the mutation that underlies the disorder would be known. That knowledge could be used as the basis for testing any other members of the family to discover those who are carriers or those who have not yet developed symptoms (presymptomatic individuals), or to determine the genetic status of fetuses. If the lab test can identify the genetic flaw that has appeared in the family, then an accurate genetic diagnosis can be made.

Complications arise when there is no information on the specific type of mutation involved, or if what looks like the same disorder can come about from mutations in any of several different genes. If the affected individual has died and there is no previously stored blood or tissue sample that can be used as the source of DNA for testing, there will be no way to know what gene is involved or exactly how the DNA had been altered. If the affected individual is alive but cannot be contacted or, if approached, is unwilling to provide a sample, this is also an impediment to direct testing. The cost of testing the affected person may also be a problem for certain consumers.

In some cases, direct testing can still proceed by looking for the most common mutations associated with the disorder. *Multiplex genetic testing,* such as is done for cystic fibrosis mutations, can search out a number of the more common mutations in the DNA. If one of these mutations is present, the direct test can discover it. If none of the common mutations are found, this reduces the likelihood that the person bears a mutant gene. However, because a rare mutation might be present, risk cannot be completely eliminated.

For several disorders, including myotonic muscular dystrophy (muscular wasting), fragile-X (mental retardation), and Huntington disease, the mutation occurs in a region of the responsible gene where groups of three bases happen to be repeated several times. For example, there may be a stretch which normally contains several repetitions of the base sequence CAG. When only a few repeats are present, there is no problem with gene function. If, instead, a mutation has occurred so that now a large number of repeats are present, gene function may be compromised. A direct test can be done to gauge the number of repeats that are there. The test can determine if the number of repeats is solidly within the normal range so that no disease will develop, or if the number is so large as to bring on the symptoms.

Though this form of direct test is typically quite straightforward, it can introduce its own set of concerns. One must be absolutely sure that the diagnosis of the affected person is correct. Even better, it would be important to establish that this person has the mutation that is the one associated with the disorder. Dr. Michael Hayden, in the Department of Medical Genetics at the University of British Columbia, has pointed out that, unless you are certain that an affected parent has the increased number of CAG repeats associated with Huntington disease, the failure to find a larger number of repeats in the offspring cannot definitively establish that they are free of risk. The problem in that family could have arisen from another neurological disorder that closely mimics Huntington disease and for which, in fact, they could be at risk. So it is important to examine the DNA of an affected family member to find out whether or not an increased number of CAG repeats is indeed present.

In Hayden's laboratory in Vancouver, they have the following policy: If they have tested the DNA from an affected relative and know for sure that the person has a gene with repeats numbering in the range that causes Huntington disease, they can tell relatives found to have repeats in the normal range on both chromosomes that they did not inherit the faulty gene. There is no chance that the genetic disease will develop. However, if no studies have been done on the individual thought to have Huntington disease, relatives who are found to have repeats in the normal range are told that there is still a very small chance—less than 1 percent—that they have inherited a genetic disorder. This is because the affected person in that family might have had some other disorder for which they may still be at risk.

Then too, there are the difficulties associated with drawing conclusions from finding a number of repeats that do not fall clearly into
either the normal or the disease range. A "gray zone" or "intermedi-
ate zone" exists between these ranges where it is not yet established
just what that number of repeats means. The question that cannot yet
be answered is: Are the number of repeats that are found capable of
actually triggering disease symptoms? With more opportunity to follow individuals whose repeat numbers fall in the gray zone, it will
eventually be possible to offer more definitive conclusions from the test.
But right now, it is not yet clear how one should interpret such results.

Direct testing can thus be relatively simple and definitive when
the diagnosis is certain and when there is already information about the
specific mutation occurring in the family, or when the changes in
the DNA are understood well enough to predict how the changed genes
function. Conversely, direct testing can be complicated and ambiguous
if there is no prior knowledge of the type of mutation that has appeared
in the family, if an affected individual cannot or will not submit to testing so that the mutation can be identified, or if scientists do not yet
know enough about particular altered forms of the genes to be sure what
the results mean.

In addition, the procedures used to analyze the DNA may themselves introduce errors that can confuse the conclusions drawn from
the test. One such error that can occur with the polymerase chain reaction procedures used in this form of direct testing might keep the gene
on one of the two chromosomes from showing up. This type of testing error could lead to the erroneous conclusion that both representatives of the gene pair are normal, when, in fact, one may possess a
mutation that yields serious health consequences.

Linkage Tests

For many genetic disorders, a direct test does not exist. Instead, the
linkage test, with its reliance on nearby DNA markers, can be used to
indicate what genes may be present. As was outlined in Chapter Two,
linkage testing is employed when the gene itself has not yet been
pinned down. It can also be used when the gene is known but is large

and contains so many different mutations that the specific mutation in a family is not identified.

Linkage testing is more elaborate and complex than direct testing. Several aspects of linkage testing distinguish it from other forms of genetic testing. These are the inescapable necessity for other family members to be involved in the testing process; the length of time that the testing can take and the costs of testing all of the family members; and problems in interpreting test results when such results can only be given as a *probability* and not as a clear-cut definitive description of the exact genetic picture. It does happen that, even after much time, effort, and money has been expended, testing yields inconclusive results. These extra demands and intricacies of linkage testing have proven to be very important considerations to consumers, as they have weighed the merits of this type of testing.

Involving the Family System.   "Why can't you just test me? What do you mean I have to get my aunt and mother and brother?" Comments like these are often heard in genetic clinics when linkage testing is discussed. Other members of the family are a vital part of the linkage testing process. They have to be included in order to establish, as firmly as possible, with what marker DNA sequences the target gene is linked in that particular family.

The number of family members who need to participate, in addition to the individual who may be seeking genetic information, differs according to the pattern of inheritance exhibited by the disorder and depending on whether it is carrier, presymptomatic, or prenatal information that is being sought. One absolute requirement for establishing the relationship between the marker site and the flawed gene is that a blood sample be available from at least one affected individual and, for some disorders, two affected individuals. Previously stored DNA or blood samples can be used for this purpose. Samples from other family members are also necessary. When two flawed genes must be present together to bring on the disorder, as in autosomal recessive inheritance, testing generally focuses on just the nuclear family. When a single copy of a flawed gene can by itself bring on the disorder, as in autosomal dominant or X-linked patterns, then cooperation of members of the extended family system is required. Depending on the situation, the testing laboratory could request blood samples from parents, siblings, grandparents, aunts, uncles, and cousins.

The main barrier to initiating linkage testing has been the problem of getting the necessary samples from family members. The difficulties are legion. The affected individual (or other family members needed for the testing) may have died. Relatives may be located at great distances—one family was dispersed across three continents. Parts of the family may have fallen out of touch through divorce and remarriage, making it hard to track them down and awkward, when they are finally reached, to have to reveal sensitive medical information. Quite often, these obstacles have discouraged any further attempt to do testing.

Even when they are approached, some family members may not wish to provide the needed blood sample. Parents of one child with Duchenne muscular dystrophy refused to allow a blood sample to be drawn. The child had been stuck so many times and was so terrified of needles that the parents did not want to subject him to anything that was not absolutely necessary for his own care. Another family, opposed to abortion, refused to allow their affected child's blood to be drawn. They were afraid that their relative might use the information to terminate a pregnancy. A young man, seeking to determine his own carrier status, was frustrated in his attempts to use linkage testing when his parents declined to contribute blood for testing. They didn't want to know which of the two of them was, as they put it, "to blame for bringing the gene into the family." There was no way a woman trying to do testing for neurofibromatosis could explain to her elderly grandmother, who refused to believe that there were such things as genes, why her blood sample was so important. Requests have been rebuffed by relatives for reasons originating in ancient family quarrels, as well as in newly resolved personal preferences about keeping one's own genetic makeup completely private.

The issue of obligation to others—particularly one's own family—is not new to moral inquiry. Modern-day ethics has placed a major emphasis on respecting the *autonomy* of the individual, on endorsing the freedom of individuals to decide for themselves what actions they choose to undertake or allow. Transferred to the medical setting, the autonomy principle means that it is up to each person, free from coercion, to decide what is done to his or her body. Even simple procedures to obtain DNA, such as having a blood sample drawn or scraping cells from the inside of the cheek, cannot be performed without the permission of the individual whose body will be invaded in order to collect the sample.

There are those who argue that individual autonomy should not be allowed to override the opportunity to achieve a benefit for others, especially in situations in which the benefits more than outweigh any harm that would be done. However, individual decisions are generally overruled only when it can be established that the person making the decision is not mentally competent either because of youth, mental retardation, or mental deterioration. Medical professionals will not be able to take a sample, no matter how important it is for linkage testing, unless permission is expressly given. The methods available to encourage other family members to provide samples are those of discussion and persuasion. Medical geneticists are willing to assist by providing explanations and details of the testing—by mail or by phone—if they are asked to do so. If these methods fail, then the linkage testing cannot be carried out.

Duration and Costs of Testing.   Even if all of the individuals needed for the linkage testing are willing to participate, making necessary arrangements can be a very complicated and time-consuming business. If the testing is part of a research study, then there will be a genetic professional assigned that responsibility. When the testing is not part of a research study, but is instead a clinically offered service, then it is the obligation of the family itself to take on many of these tasks. The logistics can be daunting. Those who have undergone this form of testing report that what works best is to have a coordinator, someone from within the family who acts as "mission control." This family member needs to make contact with the others, needs to arrange for the drawing of the blood samples, and needs to see to it that the samples are sent off to the proper place.

The time that all the sample gathering can take depends upon individual circumstances. For some, it is only a matter of a few weeks; for others, it takes months. The potential length of this initial phase frequently rules out its use in conducting prenatal testing for an already pregnant woman when no previous studies have been carried out in the family.

There is yet another waiting period: the interval from the time the samples are sent off until the time the results are reported back. Again, this waiting period varies with circumstances. It depends on the features of the disorder, on the number of family members involved, and on any requests for additional samples that may come from the laboratory. Generally, especially for commercial laboratories, this can be a week or two. However, for one young man trying to get presymptomatic testing for the Huntington disease gene, and for a woman trying to determine whether she was a carrier of the Duchenne muscular dystrophy gene, it took a year for the results to come back. (This was during the period in which linkage was the only way to test for those genes.) Even when prior linkage testing has set the stage for prenatal testing, occasional problems can occur in processing the fetal cells, and this can produce a delay in obtaining the results.

The wait can be very stressful. According to one couple having prenatal testing for spinal muscular atrophy, "It was a horrible time, you know, the time you have to wait and wonder." Another couple reported that awaiting linkage test results was "very anxiety provoking. We were hanging on pins and needles. . . . Even though the situation itself wasn't frantic, wasn't life and death, *we* were frantic." One woman, recalling the waiting period, summarized her experience in just three words: "fret, fret, fret." Indeed, because of the number of family members who may have given blood samples, the feeling of apprehension can extend across the entire family. Dr. Barbara Quinton, of the Howard University School of Medicine, has described the effect as one of "an entire family holding its breath."

Beyond the psychological burdens, there may be substantial

financial burdens incurred when carrying out the linkage studies. For those who are participating in research studies, all the costs of genetic testing are borne by the investigators. But, once the test becomes routinely available, the costs are then paid by the consumers. Most laboratories will charge a fee for each individual person so that each one receives a bill. A few laboratories have a policy of charging all testing to one account, so that the person seeking the genetic information will receive a single bill that covers all of the family testing. Presently, the charge for each individual test is about three hundred dollars. Prenatal testing can be higher if one includes the costs of chorionic villus sampling or amniocentesis. Overall costs may be several thousand dollars.

When consumers with health insurance coverage have turned to their insurance companies for assistance, they have found that the providers have different policies when it comes to covering the costs of linkage testing. Most of those having health insurance have reported few problems; in one way or another, the companies have paid for most or all of the tests. One problem area has been the refusal by some insurance companies to pay for any testing of nonaffected family members because it is not "medically indicated," even though these people are key to any interpretation of linkage relationships. Another problem has been the preference of health plans to pay for genetic testing of pregnant women but not to pay for testing prior to pregnancy. Given the time it can take to obtain the requisite samples, the obligation under some health plans to wait until a pregnancy is underway can make it difficult, if not impossible, for linkage testing to be carried out.

Many genetic counselors have felt it necessary to intervene directly with the insurance payers to explain why it is important to have testing done prior to pregnancy and why samples from unaffected as well as affected individuals are required. It is often a frustrating enterprise: Explanations painstakingly given to an employee in one division of the company are not transmitted to, or are poorly understood by, the branch with the final authority to make the decision. A crazy quilt of policies has resulted, making it difficult for consumers to determine just what genetic testing costs will be covered. To avoid the hassle—or to keep private the fact that a test was conducted—some people pay for the tests out of their own pockets.

For those who have no health insurance, the cost can be the barrier that rules out linkage testing even when it is desired. It is not only the costs of the testing itself (though these are sufficiently high to dissuade some), but other demands on the family finances can enter the picture also. If there are already affected children in the household, mothers (and occasionally fathers) have had to give up outside employment to stay home to provide constant care when it is needed, markedly lowering family income. Expenses for medicine and special equipment may stretch family finances to the breaking point. A few families were able to turn to national foundations or local charities for assistance; some chose to substitute other kinds of medical tests—ones that might be less accurate but were more affordable.

Interpreting the Test Results.   The reason any of us undergo a medical test is to find out what is, or is not, taking place in our body. People who have genetic testing are no different. They want to find out, from the testing, whether a particular gene or genetic combination is present that has implications for their immediate or long-term health. Based on their experience with other types of tests, they expect that they will get a definitive "yes or no" answer.

But contrary to this expectation, linkage testing does not, indeed cannot, provide an absolutely sure conclusion. As discussed in Chapter Two, the test result obtained is not given as a definite answer one way or the other, but is expressed as a probability—the chance or odds that a gene (or a pair of genes) has been inherited. Like the man looking for his car keys under a lamppost, not because that's where he dropped the keys but because that's where the light is better, linkage testing depends on the light shed by marker sequences in the DNA to gain a sense of what is happening in the nearby target gene which is hidden from view.

The DNA from blood samples of family members who participate in the testing helps establish what markers are present and what forms of the gene they are linked with in each family. The test then draws *mathematical* conclusions about whether the flawed gene or genes are present by looking for the markers present in the person or fetus for whom the testing is being carried out. There is no guarantee that the markers and the genes will stay permanently linked together. There is always the possibility that markers have been switched during the normal processes of "crossing over" that can occur anywhere on the chromosomes during sperm and egg formation. The possibility that a switch-over has occurred limits the degree of assurance with which you can draw conclusions from any linkage test. The closer the marker is to the gene, the higher the degree of assurance. This is because gene-to-marker proximity makes it less likely that a switch-over has occurred on the short stretch of chromosome in between marker and gene. Also, if there are markers on both sides of the target gene, any rearrangement of these flanking markers makes it easier to determine if a switch-over has occurred.

Linkage test results are thus given as a probability, based on the likelihood that marker and target gene have remained together. So the report that comes back from the laboratory is not stated as a definitive finding, but instead is stated as the probability that the gene combination is present. For example, the consumer may be informed that there is a 95 percent chance that she is a carrier; but a small (5 percent or one-in-twenty) chance still remains that she is not. A test result giving a 92 percent chance that the fetus will be unaffected means that 8 percent of the time the child will be found to be affected after birth. Although we all take chances when making life's important decisions, we don't normally think in terms of probabilities. Probabilities are difficult for people to interpret and deal with.

Recent progress in genetic science has greatly expanded the number of markers available for use in linkage testing. Some markers are located on the chromosome at positions extremely close to, or even within, the target gene. In such cases, the probability that the test correctly predicts the actual genes present will be quite high. For the less well known areas of the chromosome—or where there are no markers flanking the target gene—the probability of a correct prediction is lower.

When considering linkage testing, consumers are forced to confront the reality that a test result that seems almost a sure thing in some cases just is not. "It makes me nervous," said a woman faced with the prospect of linkage testing, "I worry. But I don't have any choice." "That's the way of the world," said another, "Nothing is perfect. There are no guarantees in life."

Studies were done, in the early days of linkage testing, to assess what degree of discrepancy (between what the linkage test predicts and what the actual genetic status of the person is) was acceptable to consumers. Most of the people surveyed indicated that they would not accept a linkage test if discrepancies occurred more than 10 percent of the time. A 1 percent rate of disagreement was considered acceptable. Many of those I interviewed for this book were in substantial agreement with these figures. Said one mother having prenatal testing for spinal muscular atrophy, "If there is a 98 percent or 99 percent chance of rain, you get out an umbrella."

Nevertheless, attitudes toward risk differ widely. There are people who have a bottle of wine with dinner and those who are teetotalers; there are joggers and couch potatoes; there are fast-food fanatics and health-food aficionados. Some individuals are willing to use a test even if the chance of getting a wrong result is higher than 10 percent. As one woman stated when faced with prenatal testing for SMA, "If the test could give me a 90 percent or 80 percent chance of having a healthy baby, that would be better than the 75 percent chance I now have using the Mendelian ratios [the risk figures calculated from the standard inheritance patterns]." And for one man thinking about presymptomatic testing for a late-onset disorder, even coming away with a 51 percent chance that he would be spared would be good enough.

With all the markers now available, and the opportunity, where there are flanking markers, to determine if linkage relationships have been altered by a cross-over event, the accuracy of the predictions provided can be quite high. The chance of an incorrect conclusion may be less than 5 percent, or even, for some portions of the chromosome, less than 1 percent. Still, those reflecting on this form of genetic testing have to consider the small chance that the prediction can turn out to be wrong. One woman whose son was born with Duchenne muscular dystrophy after the linkage test had shown that there was a 95 percent chance that he would not be affected, pointed out that everyone takes a chance with any pregnancy that the child will be born with some kind of serious problem.

Occasionally, it does happen that, despite everyone's best efforts, the testing laboratory will not be able to provide any useful results. They will be unable to draw any conclusions at all. The official term for this is "noninformative." A noninformative outcome occurs when it is not possible to determine which marker is traveling with the flawed gene in a family. This outcome can also occur if it turns out that the same marker is associated with both the flawed gene and its normal counter-part, so that the two different genes cannot be distinguished from each other. "It seems to me it would be a lot to go through and still not have answers," said one woman who opted against having prenatal linkage testing for Coffin-Lowry syndrome.

With the increasing number of markers that are useful for linkage testing, noninformativeness is decreasing as a linkage-test complica-tion. But it can still occur. When it does, it often evokes considerable anger and bitterness—the disappointment intensified by all the effort and expense that had been invested in the attempt to gain genetic infor-mation. "A waste of time," was the reaction of an irate consumer. "How could you do this to me?" shouted another. One couple, after the death of their infant, were tested to see if the markers on their chromo-some would permit them to do prenatal testing at the next pregnancy. When they learned that their markers were such that the test would be noninformative, they were left to wonder, "Can anything possibly go right?" The psychological pain from such dashed hopes can be as severe as what occurs when an informative linkage-test result yields a high-risk prognosis.

The deficiencies of linkage testing can sometimes be overcome. Improvements in the test can allow a previously noninformative situ-ation to become informative. The participation of additional relatives may provide the needed information for determining the way the target gene and DNA marker are linked together. Additionally, it may take the discovery of specific mutations and the appearance of a direct test to clarify the genetic picture. When a direct test for Huntington disease became available in 1993, most of those who were first in line to use it had been frustrated earlier in their attempts to use linkage testing. The direct test now offered them a chance, at last, to gain the information they sought. Interestingly, genetic counselors working with Huntington disease families have noted that, of those for whom linkage testing had been informative, few who had received a low-risk prognosis asked to be retested with the new direct test. Apparently they remain satisfied with the relatively high probability that their linkage-test result is correct. Thus they decide to pass up the direct test, even though it would yield a definite result eliminating the need to worry about the low (but not zero) probability of an incorrect linkage-test prognosis.

In Chapter Seven, I discuss the rate of recent scientific progress in moving from a linked marker to the identification of the gene itself. This rate is used as a rough guide for how soon we may expect linkage testing to be replaced by direct testing. There is no assurance that direct testing will ever become possible or practical for all disorders. Linkage testing may be the only testing procedure in many situations: when the genes involved are very large or difficult to work with; where, instead of a few commonly shared mutations, the mutations are unique to each family; and for those individuals with quite unusual changes in their DNA.

The Timing

The number of genetic tests now available, and the surge of new tests expected from intensive research efforts such as the Human Genome Project (described in Chapter Seven), have created a general expectation that consumers will eagerly climb aboard a testing bandwagon and insist on having the tests done as a matter of course. Most consumers interviewed, however, are considerably more restrained in their enthusiasm for genetic testing and approach it with caution. For them, the availability of testing is not the point. Instead, the main point for consumers is whether or not the information testing can provide comes both *in* time and *at* a time when it can help to guide future family planning or health-care decisions. If the overall timing is right, then this may impel them to proceed with testing. If it is not, then testing tends to be regarded as serving no practical purpose and, consequently, as better off postponed or not worth pursuing at all.

TESTING TIMELINE

The element of timing enters the decision process in a very immediate way. Since most people first become aware of the availability of genetic testing during the course of an ongoing pregnancy, the time window for performing the testing and getting results back may be quite short. The legal limit for carrying out an abortion represents one possible time constraint. Different considerations cause some women to be reluctant to undergo amniocentesis for genetic testing of the fetal cells. Since amniocentesis is done nearly midway through a pregnancy, it carries a small risk of terminating the pregnancy. These women do not want to add any risk, even the small risk associated with fetal cell collection using this method, to a pregnancy that has progressed that far. The "window of opportunity" for testing can be quite brief. As noted above, when linkage testing is used, doing the required genetic tests of family members and collecting the fetal cell sample may take considerable time. The later into a pregnancy the testing starts, the greater the possibility that time will run out in the quest for genetic information.

Sometimes the time pressure that is felt has less to do with the realities of the testing process than it does with the building up of a profound sense of urgency—an urgency exacerbated by the sheer weariness that becomes a fact of life for parents already caring for an ill infant. One couple attributed their decision to start linkage testing, within weeks of the birth of a daughter with spinal muscular atrophy, to the fact that they were going through a period in which they were living on pure emotion. From exhaustion and grief, they were not thinking clearly. They have never regretted having had the testing, though they now, in retrospect, question why it all had to be done in such a hurry.

Unlike the severe time crunch for genetic testing during pregnancy, the time period during which genetic testing can be done for disorders of late onset can be considerable—months, years, even decades. Individuals who want to know whether or not they will develop a disorder later in life have the opportunity to rely first on some of the nongenetic tests from the host of diagnostic tools in the medical arsenal. There are all manner of medical tests that can search out early signs of malfunction associated with a disorder. Testing for specific blood factors, for muscle or other tissue components, and for bone or organ architecture, may be carried out. The relative simplicity and low cost of these techniques make them desirable for many consumers, and allow consideration of genetic testing to be deferred. Even when genetic tests are sought, there is usually no feeling of having to race to conclude the testing process.

AGE AND STAGE-OF-LIFE

An oft-cited reason for lack of interest in carrier testing is the decision not to have any children (or any more children). Having genetic information would not change anything for many of these people. Though she would be "running to the door to take the test if she wanted more children," one mother of a child with an X-linked disorder has decided not to have any more. For her, testing to see if she is a carrier would be an unnecessary activity. For a mother of a boy with Duchenne muscular dystrophy, the cost of the test to see if she is a carrier is just not worth it when she and her husband have found that they lack the physical and emotional strength to deal with any more children in their household. Identifying the precise mutation or the linkage pattern could satisfy one's curiosity, but consumers usually see this as insufficient justification for testing if they are not interested in having more children.

When a child has been born with a rare disorder associated with a recessive gene, there is often a strong belief among relatives in the extended family that there is no need for carrier testing. Even if they turned out to be a carrier, they reason, it would be very unlikely for their spouse (who is not a blood relation) to bear a defect in the same recessive gene. Thus it would be very unlikely that their children could have the disorder. Statistics, based on our current knowledge of the frequencies of mutations, certainly do favor such a conclusion. However, it happens to be the case that two of the families who participated in my study were very unlucky in just this way: The unrelated partner bore a mutation located in the very same gene—a fact made apparent when an affected child was born.

For parents who have an affected child and who want to have more children, the genetic test provides the opportunity to verify their own carrier status and to undertake prenatal genetic studies. Some surveys indicated, for families with a child having cystic fibrosis, an overall lack of interest in genetic testing. However, many medical geneticists have noted that a majority of such families *still intending to have more children* do make use of prenatal testing at subsequent pregnancies. The decision to have a prenatal test opens the issue of aborting if the fetus is found to be affected. But even in the case of such a diagnosis, some parents decide to continue the pregnancy. This is discussed below in the section called "The Options."

Prenatal testing is done to obtain genetic information about the health (and future health) of the fetus. The parents are the sole decision makers for this type of testing. What about testing others in the family? The siblings of a child affected with a recessive disorder may be carriers of the gene for that disorder. Genetic testing can determine who among the healthy sisters and brothers are carriers. The children of a parent with a dominant disorder of late onset may have inherited that same gene. Genetic testing can identify a child who has inherited a gene whose effects are not yet discernible.

Is childhood the right time to perform genetic tests? This is a question that continues to arouse a great deal of emotion and controversy. The emphasis on individual autonomy in our culture translates to the importance of permitting each and every person to determine just *what* genetic information he or she wants to receive, and *when.*

There is no universal agreement among physicians, geneticists, ethicists, or testing laboratories about when this autonomy begins and what might be the appropriate age to have children tested. Each genetic service center has formulated its own standards and conditions—and the policies differ. The suggested minimum age for testing ranges from eighteen years down to eleven or twelve. A Presidential Commission in 1982 offered the view that children fourteen years or older could be considered competent to consent to personal health-care decisions. In 1994, another panel, the Committee on Assessing Genetic Risks of the Institute of Medicine, put forth the following recommendation:

> Children should generally be tested only for genetic disorders
> for which there exists an effective curative or preventive treat-
> ment that must be instituted early in life to achieve maximum
> benefit. Childhood testing is not appropriate for carrier status,
> untreatable childhood diseases, and late-onset diseases that
> cannot be prevented or forestalled by early treatment.

Thus, in the absence of an immediate need for the information, this state-ment warns against genetic testing of children. Testing should be postponed until a child has reached an age when he or she can reason-ably consent to the testing procedure. The Institute of Medicine com-mittee members were concerned about psychological harm to children, such as possible damage to their self-esteem, and were distinctly uneasy about carrier testing carried out prior to the age of eighteen.

Others who have looked at this issue prefer a sliding scale for test-ing, depending on the usefulness of the genetic information in guiding health-care interventions and reproductive decisions, with fifteen as the minimum age for testing. Drawing on the experience gathered in sickle-cell gene testing programs, and recognizing the trend toward earlier sexual activity by adolescents, still others feel that testing should be available from age twelve. Dr. Robert F. Murray, Jr., of the Howard University School of Medicine, supports moving the minimum suggested age down to the preteen years. These young people, he believes, are learning about biology in their science classes and may understand genetics better than many adults. There is an additional value in having them think about the significance of becoming parents, and what the possibilities are for having a child who might be sick or who might require special life-long attention.

Some experienced genetic professionals believe that, in individual circumstances, it may actually be preferable to test children for carrier status in advance of their adolescent years, even children as young as six. This is often a calmer stage of life—less beset with the complications and conflicts so frequently apparent during the teens. Testing during this early period avoids intensifying the teenage fear of finding oneself different from one's peers. Information acquired early on, they claim, can be more readily accepted. Any decision to do carrier testing early has to be made on a case-by-case basis. However, these same professionals also stress that for presymptomatic testing, when there is no way to *modify* the course of the disorder associated with the gene (most notably, for Huntington disease), testing should be deferred until the person is mature enough to deal with the implications of such testing.

During the course of the interviews that form the basis of this book, parents were asked about their views on testing children to determine whether or not they are carriers. Most of these parents indicated that they preferred to wait until their children were older before filling them in on the details of the family's genetic history and bringing up the possibility of genetic testing. When would they bring this up? For these parents it was when their offspring were of child-bearing age, particularly if they were in a serious relationship and thinking about getting married. There were many reasons offered for waiting until late adolescence or beyond. "I don't feel *I* want to know until then," asserted one parent whose daughter could be a carrier for an X-linked disorder. "For now, I try not to think about it." Several parents noted that their older teenage children were beset with school and other problems. They did not want to add new worries to their children's problems. And one parent was concerned that his children, who were in the midst of competing for college scholarships, might be turned down if they were found to be carriers.

When genetic information has already been obtained in the course of testing the family, as happens in linkage testing, parents have to determine when the time is right to share that result. Should the result be shared immediately or would it be better to wait until the child is older? Most of the parents consulted in this study have decided not to offer any information unless they are asked. One ten-year-old asked her dad, while they were both watching a science program on public television, what the results were of her test for the Duchenne muscular dystrophy gene. Taken aback, he gulped and said simply, "You are a carrier." "That's what I thought," she said, before giving her rapt attention back to the program. If the fateful question never arises, parents are faced with deciding when to bring it up. All the same arguments offered in the controversy about the best time for testing children apply. here as well. What all sides agree on is that there is no one absolutely right time to tell children. It will always be a difficult call.

The Options

In Robert Frost's famous poem "The Road Not Taken," a traveler standing at a fork in the trail is faced with deciding which path to take. Proceeding on one path will be certain to bring some new pleasures and challenges, but it will also lead him away from whatever pleasures and challenges would have awaited him on the other path. No matter which he picks, there are bound to be some gains and there will be some losses. Which way should he go? In a real sense, those faced with a decision about genetic testing are presented with a similar choice. A genetic test can provide information that opens up new vistas and opportunities, at the same time that it inevitably shuts out others. The other pathway, that of not having the test, brings its own assortment of pluses and minuses. Understanding and sorting through the options— as well as they can be known or guessed at in advance—are key components in deciding how useful a genetic test would be.

PRENATAL TESTING

Hidden from view and not visible until the very moment of birth, the developing fetus has always been the source of speculation. Will it be a boy or a girl? Will all the fingers and toes be there? Will it be healthy? The veil of mystery surrounding these questions began to be pushed away as medical and genetic technologies—such as ultrasound studies and the improved procedures for examining fetal chromosomes—

gave the first glimmers of information about the status of the developing fetus. DNA testing dramatically expands this opportunity, allowing information about the presence or absence of many different types of single-gene disorders to be revealed well before the time of birth.

Prenatal genetic testing usually becomes of interest when there is a known risk that the fetus could inherit genes which contribute to the onset of a disorder. If one of the parents has a dominantly inherited disorder, or is found to be a carrier of an X-linked disorder, the gene in question can be transmitted to offspring. If both parents carry the same recessive gene that is associated with a disorder, then future children may be at risk for the disorder. The degree of that risk can be calculated from the pattern of inheritance: dominant, recessive, or X-linked. Testing of fetal DNA can help parents go beyond these pen-and-paper risk calculations and obtain a more precise snapshot of the genes of the fetus.

The discovery that the fetus has *not* inherited a genetic complement that can result in a disorder (or that the probability of that occurrence is low) is a great relief. This is what all parents hope they will hear. However, the test results may come back otherwise. One woman who sought prenatal genetic testing for spinal muscular atrophy after losing a child to the disease advised, "The important question to keep in mind is: What are you going to do if the test doesn't go your way?" If that happens, then a new choice appears. The parents can elect to terminate the pregnancy or, alternatively, they can prepare for the birth of a child who will be born with or who will later develop some type of health problem.

Few issues arouse as much controversy and passionate disagreement as does the issue of abortion. The same wide spectrum of opinion that characterizes our society at large was present among the participants in this interview study. On occasion, even husband and wife had widely differing views. But making a decision in which abortion is an option is not like choosing sides in a debate carried on from a soapbox or at a political rally. It becomes a deeply personal struggle. Even for women whose moral or religious beliefs are consistent with permitting pregnancy termination, or who consider themselves solidly "pro-choice," the thought of possibly terminating a pregnancy is deeply troubling. "It was a choice between terrible and awful. Watching a bright, alert, happy baby die is terrible and abortion is awful," said one woman. Another woman, the mother of a boy with Duchenne muscular dystrophy, described her anxiety during the period of testing for that disorder at her next pregnancy. She was approaching her twentieth week of the pregnancy and was emotionally bonded to the fetus. She was starting to look pregnant, and many of her good friends knew she was pregnant. She kept thinking how much she loved the son she already had and recalling what a joy he had been as a baby. It would have been very hard to terminate the new pregnancy. She and her husband sought both genetic and psychological counseling during this time to help them think matters through. As it turned out, the test showed that the fetus did not inherit the mutation for Duchenne muscular dystrophy. Since then, she has decided not to have any more children because she does not want to have to go through that distressing decision-making dilemma again.

Many couples who find abortion an unacceptable option feel that the test is unnecessary. They elect to wait and see what happens. But others, equally opposed to pregnancy termination, wish to have a genetic test so that they gain the gift of time. If it turns out that the fetus is affected, they feel the advance warning will give them more time to move beyond their initial reaction and to make preparations that can best meet the needs of the child. Such plans could include identifying medical specialists in their region and getting ready to deal with possible complications. The plans may also include finding out what relevant educational and community services are available, and reorganizing personal and work schedules to fit in the anticipated needs of the new child with those of the rest of the family.

When confronting actual, not theoretical, events, several consumers have reexamined and revised their views about prenatal testing and, for some, the acceptability of abortion. Changes of opinion have gone both ways. For example, one woman had twice selected pregnancy termination based on test results which indicated that a disorder would develop. For her third pregnancy, she decided not to use any prenatal testing at all. She had come to feel that it would be too painful to go through another abortion, concluding, "It is better to have a baby for a couple of months than not to have it at all." Another woman had, in the past, been opposed to any form of testing. Reflecting on the needs of her ill child, she has decided that testing would be the route she would now elect to follow, since both she and her husband feel that they do not want "to have another child suffer." Another couple changed their previous anti-abortion stance when they determined that it would be impossible for them to take on the responsibility of caring for another affected child.

The pros and cons of the abortion question are not the only issues consumers bring into a decision about prenatal testing. For many, the inability of the DNA tests to tell from the genes that are present just when the symptoms will appear, or how mild or severe the disorder will turn out to be, is an important drawback. The effect on the family, particularly on the other children, is also an issue. One mother of a son who has cystic fibrosis has rejected any attempt at prenatal testing. She explains that she would never want her son to think that she didn't love him or give him any reason to imagine that she regretted he had been born.

Some genetic professionals believe that, in the future, it may not be the health of the fetus but of the grandchildren—that is, the fetus's potential children—that could become part of the testing decision for some. This could arise with a disorder such as myotonic muscular dystrophy, where children of affected females are at risk for developing the more serious early-onset form. It could also arise with fragile-X mental retardation, in which unaffected carrier-female fetuses could produce eggs with the full-blown mutation, putting the fetus's potential male children at risk. However, this sort of consideration (effects on potential grandchildren) was never mentioned by any of the consumers interviewed.

CARRIER TESTING

Until recently, carriers of flawed, recessive genes have been unaware of the presence of these genes in themselves. In fact, it would be very difficult or impossible for them to know this because, in carriers, the normal gene masks the presence of the flawed gene and protects the individual against harmful effects. It is only when no functional dominant gene is present in the gene pair that difficulties can occur. Such unmasking can occur during reproduction if both partners happen to be carriers of the same flawed gene and if, by chance (25 percent of the time, in this situation), the sperm or egg that each contributes in fertilization contains the recessive gene. Carrier testing can allow both partners to determine if they carry the same flawed gene.

For X-linked disorders, the unmasking can result if a woman who is a carrier passes the X chromosome with the flawed gene to a male fetus. Since a male fetus has a Y chromosome as the second sex chromosome, the effects of the flawed gene will appear. Carrier testing allows families in which there is a single child with an X-linked disorder (such as Duchenne muscular dystrophy) to learn whether or not the mother is a carrier. If she is not, it means that the disorder arose from a new mutation that has altered only her son's genetic material.

Usually, if a woman who has had a child with an X-linked disorder is found not to be a carrier by DNA testing, she is cautioned that there may still be a small risk—of the order of 1 to 10 percent—that the mutation resides in some of the egg cells still present in her ovary. This is called "gonadal mosaicism." That is, a new mutation may be present in a small fraction of the cells that form the gonads—the ovary or testes—of the parents, and absent from all other tissues. If that has happened, then even when DNA extracted from blood samples yields a normal result, there remains a risk that the mutated gene exists in a few of the cells of the gonads and that it could be passed along in fertilization. It is hard to estimate such a risk.

Carrier detection, using enzyme and other biochemical tests, has been possible for some time for a few genetic conditions such as sickle-cell anemia and Tay-Sachs disease. The new DNA tests can now detect many other types of recessive genes (either by looking directly for known changes in the gene or by making predictions based on markers linked to the gene). Testing to determine carrier status may be brought to the attention of relatives of a person with a recessive genetic disorder, because genes are shared in families, and the relatives may also have inherited the gene. Increasingly, carrier testing for some of the more common genetic disorders (such as cystic fibrosis) is being offered to women during pregnancy. This is part of the growing package of available tests they can make use of, even when there is no history of the disorder in the family.

The main reason offered for considering carrier testing is to get information that could be used as the basis for reproductive planning. In the not-too-distant past, when only calculated odds were available, many siblings of a child with cystic fibrosis (who had a two-thirds risk of being a carrier) chose not to reproduce. In one report, the figure was as high as 70 percent. In the case of X-linked disorders, women who did not know if they were carriers had to consider whether they should have children. One option was to terminate all pregnancies in which the fetus was found to be male, since any carrier's son would have a 50 percent probability of having the disorder. If through testing they could *know* whether or not they carried the recessive gene, they would be spared this predicament. And, of course, a woman who learned that she was not a carrier of an X-linked disorder would now no longer need to be fearful of having a son.

For some individuals who had genetic testing, results that showed they were not carriers were accompanied by a phenomenon they had not expected—sibling guilt. Finding oneself spared while others in the family are still faced with potential genetic problems can be an uncomfortable and cheerless situation. One teenager who has two brothers with an X-linked disorder wanted desperately for the test to show that she was a carrier, so that she would fit in with her brothers and her mother. In another family, the sister who turned out not to be a carrier of the X-linked recessive gene was the one who had the greatest problem accepting the testing results.

Finding out that one is a carrier provides information about risks associated with future pregnancies. It can be an aid in making reproductive decisions and opens up the option of using prenatal testing. A woman who learns that she is a carrier of an X-linked recessive gene knows that her future male children would have a 50 percent chance of having the disorder, while her daughters would have a 50 percent chance of being carriers like herself. (Like herself, her carrier daughters would be healthy, displaying no signs of genetic illness.) For this woman, DNA testing yields a result with direct implications for future pregnancies.

The use of carrier testing for reproductive decisions is not always so straightforward for the non-X-linked recessive disorders—conditions caused by genes that are not on the X chromosome but are located on any of the other 22 chromosome pairs, known as the autosomes. For these autosomal recessive genes, both partners would have to be carriers for there to be any risk to their offspring. If both are carriers, then at each pregnancy there is a 25 percent probability that the fetus would be affected.

For a known carrier to determine whether there is any chance of having an affected child, the next step would be to have DNA testing to see if the partner is also a carrier. There can be some problems making this assessment. If linkage testing is the method used, then the desired carrier information could only be obtained if the partner's family happens to have a history of the disorder, allowing it to be genetically tracked. If there is no history in the partner's family, linkage testing is no help. Even if direct DNA testing can be used, it may not be possible to determine the partner's carrier status unambiguously, because testing negative for any of the common mutations cannot rule out the presence of the rare mutations that the test does not detect. However, ruling out the common mutations does significantly reduce the likelihood of being a carrier and, therefore, the reproductive risk.

Once testing indicates that someone is a carrier, another decision point arises. Others in the family may also have inherited the same gene. Should they be told? Is there an obligation to share genetic news with others once it has been obtained? How should this be communicated? Could it be postponed if family members are preoccupied with personal or other problems? The privacy of one's own personal genetic information cannot be preserved when other family members are informed of the possibility of a risk.

Dr. Marcus Pembrey, at the Institute of Child Health in London, points to the importance of family ties and the accompanying societal expectation that family members will take care to look after each other's interests. In general, part of this family responsibility involves making important information—including genetic information—available to one another. Many scholars who have looked at this issue concur. Based on her study of the legal, ethical, and sociological sources, Lori Andrews, a legal scholar and medical ethicist, has summarized it this way: Though there is no legal duty, "there is a moral duty to share genetic information with a relative if that information could be beneficial to the relative."

There is also a broad consensus that the person who has undergone genetic counseling or had genetic tests should be responsible for transmitting information about potential risk to others in the family. Genetic professionals have a firm commitment to the privacy of their interaction with the consumer and to the confidentiality of genetic information. It is one of the fundamental tenets of their professional codes and is regarded as a necessary condition for establishing and maintaining bonds of trust with their clients. Except for those very rare circumstances in which revealing information may prevent some immediate and grave harm to others, they will neither initiate contact with family members nor divulge to them the results of genetic tests that have already been carried out. Legal traditions surrounding medical practice support this stance. As discussed in Chapter Three, genetic counselors and other genetic professionals are willing to assist by providing written material and responding to questions if they are contacted by family members who have already been alerted.

Consumers report a broad range of reactions when notifying relatives. One group of sisters, learning that they could be carriers of a gene for an X-linked disorder, went for counseling as a group. Some of them later chose to have testing and, again, they went together to get the results. The testing process brought the whole family closer together. In another case, the reaction was different. When the parent of a child newly diagnosed with cystic fibrosis broached this subject with the family, it was awkward. "It caused a big hullabaloo. Now I am always the grim reaper and I rain on everybody's parade because I am a reminder of what could happen." Others found that distance and strained relationships inhibited any communication or made it a practical impossibility. Sometimes members of the family were unavailable, unapproachable, or unwilling to listen. The news, when given, was poorly understood by some and perceived as threatening. One woman's mother-in-law refused to speak to her for a year.

The lesson learned from the earliest carrier screening programs (such as were carried out for sickle-cell anemia and Tay-Sachs disease), and still observed today, is that lack of understanding of what it means to be a carrier can provoke unfortunate personal reactions. Psychological distress and problems with self-image are common. Similar lack of understanding by others, including insurance companies and potential employers, has led to some forms of social stigmatization. (These issues are discussed in more detail in Chapter Six.) Among the interviewees for this book, however, no one reported any problems like these.

PRESYMPTOMATIC TESTING

As we have seen in Chapter Two, disorders can be attributed to faulty dominant genes, which exert their effects when present in a single dose. Sometimes these dominant genes do not immediately reveal their presence. It may take years, even decades, before the kinds of physical or biochemical changes they produce are observed. Disorders showing a late-onset pattern include myotonic muscular dystrophy, adult polycystic kidney disease, Huntington disease, and some forms of retinitis pigmentosa.

In the past, people who had a 50 percent risk for developing such a genetic disorder because they had an affected parent would only know whether they had inherited the critical gene when the first signs or symptoms appeared. Until that happened, they were frequently faced with a great deal of uncertainty. Often, they vacillated back and forth on a daily basis, sometimes seeing themselves as being risk free and sometimes seeing themselves as certain to have inherited the disorder. Because the age of onset can vary, they could not feel sure, until very late in their lives, that they had not inherited the gene. It is easy to see how this type of uncertainty could create emotional distress and complicate attempts to make plans for the future concerning marriage, family, education, and career. The advent of new forms of genetic testing has changed this picture. For many of the disorders in question, looking for the telltale signs of the mutation in the DNA can now serve as a kind of genetic crystal ball. The presence of these signs indicates that the faulty gene has been inherited from an affected parent. Moreover, testing can be performed at any time in advance of when symptoms would first show up, even during the prenatal period.

Most people who proceed along the pathway of presymptomatic testing give as their main reason the wish to replace uncertainty with a firm indication, one way or the other, about their genetic status. They want to use that information to make plans for their future, and they look forward to the stability of knowing, rather than the experience of endless doubt and continual self-searching for signals that the disorder is developing. When DNA tests became available for Huntington disease in 1986, it was expected that a large fraction of people at risk would seek out the testing for these very reasons. In reality, the actual percentage who chose testing was quite small, about 10 percent.

One woman, who had lost her mother to Huntington disease and whose two siblings already showed signs of the disease, exemplifies part of the reason for this lower-than-expected response rate. She was very excited when she first heard of the test. But the more she thought about it, the less convinced she was that it was right for her. The test, she decided, was a double-edged sword. It could tell her that she *had* the gene, but couldn't tell her *when* she would get the disease or *whether* her physicians could offer any treatment. As she thought further, she realized that she had gained control of the anxiety she felt. She had already come to terms with living at risk. It seemed to her that it would be better to remain uncertain than to have to deal with the new problems presented by the test results: the "sibling" or "survivor" guilt if she did not have the gene, the anxiety of waiting for the disease to develop if she did have the gene. It was preferable for her to continue, as she put it, with the "security of the uncertainty."

From studies of at-risk people, it appears that most who have opted for testing are satisfied that they finally have an answer. These studies have also found that, as the cloud of uncertainty vanishes, it is often replaced by a mixed bag of reactions and consequences, no matter what the result. A low-risk result (obtained through linkage testing) or a mutation-free result (determined by direct testing) can permit people to plan for their future without the specter of the disorder hanging over their heads. It also allows them to tell their children that they are spared concerns about having the family's genetic disorder. But many found that they now had to face up to other problems in their lives, problems that were ignored while they were focused on their genetic risk or which they wrongly attributed to genetic risk. And they had to replace long-held habits of thought. For example, a person who is convinced that life will be short may have little motivation for investing in education or career-building or in long-term human relationships. Changing these attitudes, to adjust to a normal life span, can be hard to do.

Individuals undergoing testing must face the possibility that they could come away with a high-risk result. Research studies on those at risk for Huntington disease have found that getting such a result typically brings on depression and other psychological reactions. While these reactions do abate in time, counseling and other types of emotional and social support services are definitely helpful for dealing with these problems. Many people in the high-risk group did take steps to organize various aspects of their lives, including financial ones, so that they could be better prepared at that future time when the symptoms became severe.

It is not yet known how typical these reactions are for other late-onset disorders. Retinitis pigmentosa (RP) is a disorder characterized by changes in the cells of the retina of the eye. It can lead to blindness and there is as yet no treatment. Consumers considering the possibility of presymptomatic testing for RP had mixed feelings. On the one hand, some felt that knowing in advance would be helpful for making appropriate career decisions and for developing skills that would help them cope with the impaired vision to come. On the other hand, there were those who felt that knowing in advance would cause unnecessary worry, especially in children, and that it would stunt creativity by discouraging those having the gene from getting involved in the visual arts.

Just as carrier testing can provide some family members with unexpected genetic information, presymptomatic testing may reveal to some family members information about their genetic status that they may not wish to have. For instance, if the grandchild of a person with a disorder is tested and is shown to have inherited the flawed gene, it will automatically tell the at-risk parent of that child that he or she must also have the gene. Some Huntington disease testing programs, in order to respect the desire of individuals *to not know,* will refuse to do testing unless both the at-risk parent and the at-risk child agree to the test.

Insurance companies will certainly be interested in finding out whether applicants for life or health insurance policies have a higher-than-average risk for serious, life-threatening health problems. Once a person undergoes presymptomatic genetic testing and receives a more accurate indication of the real risk that he or she faces, it will be necessary to provide that information, when asked, on insurance application forms. Some genetic advocacy groups suggest that people make insurance arrangements *before* they have testing, so that there cannot be any question of hiding information about their health situation. If one has gained genetic information, it is a misrepresentation of fact to deny that it exists. Further discussion on how much access insurance companies and employers ought to have to genetic information will be found in Chapter Six.

Making a Decision about Genetic Testing

Whether or not to have DNA testing is an important decision for oneself and, most often, for others in the family. It would be nice to have a checklist to use to weigh each of the four factors described above, to balance each one against each of the others, and to be led directly, in a step-by-step fashion, to the right decision. But there is no magic formula for making a decision of this type. There is no section at the back of the book to turn to for the right answer. There is no scoring system to tell us what category we fit into, like the one we use when filling out a magazine questionnaire.

The people who have shared their views and experiences with me made very different kinds of choices. But on one point there was strong agreement: Individuals have to make the judgment for themselves. No one else knows his or her life circumstances better and no one else will have to live with the consequences. They would not want, nor would ever accept, having anyone else impose a decision on them.

One set of parents with an ill child summarized the basis for their own decision to reject testing—a decision grounded in the realities of their day-to-day lives:

> Genetic testing is not for us. This is a hard disease to live with and we don't want to go through this again. We would not inflict this on another child. We have not had a full night's sleep in years. We are always tired and could not handle taking care of an infant again. And it would be difficult for Bobby to see another kid in the family doing things he can't do. . . . Our decision wouldn't be right for someone else. People need to make their own decisions.

A woman, on her way to have chorionic villus sampling so that a prenatal DNA test could be done on the fetus, was aghast at being confronted by a picket line of anti-abortion activists. She remembers wondering how they could offer a judgment without knowing what she and her husband had already been through and thinking angrily: "How many of you have raised a terminally ill child? Don't do this. This is my decision and I am going into it as knowledgeable as I think we could be about the consequences." Another woman who had undergone DNA testing twice, aborting the first pregnancy and then having an affected child due to a mistakenly negative result the second time, would want to have testing were she to become pregnant again. She asserted that: "Each family has to make its own decision. It has to be made individually based on how strong a family it is and how the family could deal with the disease. Government and religious groups need to stay out of it."

No prepackaged ready-made solutions exist for what is the right thing to do. Nor do perfect solutions exist. There is no "one size fits all" scenario. As on so many other important occasions, the details really matter. Strict rules or regulations are out of the question. They are too rigid. They fail to take into account individual differences, and individual differences are the hallmark of the human condition. Guidelines, while helpful, also fall short. They cease to be meaningful when the particulars of the immediate situation differ from those envisioned when the guidelines were formulated.

To test or not to test? This is an intensely personal decision. It has to fit into the landscape of one's life—a landscape that includes personal values, family realities, and human relationships. It has to fit with one's physical, emotional, and financial strengths and limitations. Those who have described their experience have emphasized that it takes great effort to sort out what to do. One couple talked it over and over, "joining both their memories and understanding to see what they knew and felt." Another consumer described the process as "a matter of struggling back and forth between yes and no until eventually we both came to a decision." There seems to be no quick and easy path.

However, the fact that each decision has to be arrived at independently does not mean that it has to be made in isolation. Many consumers have found that others have been valuable allies as they worked their way through the decision process. Most often, their physician and the genetic professional have played important roles.

That this should be so is not a surprise. What is generally termed "the physician/patient relationship" has been the bulwark of medical care since the dawn of modern medicine. The private interaction between the physician and the patient has traditionally been the locus of most medical decision making. The physician, the expert in medical matters, is expected to analyze and evaluate the relevant aspects of a situation, provide information, lay out the options, and recommend a course of action. First and foremost, the physician's goal is to do the best for the patient. In recent years, the patient (or consumer) has played a much more active role in this relationship. The patient has taken on responsibility for selecting the most acceptable course of action from among the possibilities of treatment. This includes refusing any proposed treatment. This cooperative model is currently under attack, battered by pressures pushing the physician to contain health-care costs by limiting access to tests and services. This is unfortunate, because a physician's sensitivity and responsiveness to individual needs and preferences, in an atmosphere of trust, is important. It allows the physician/patient relationship, and by extension the genetic counselor/consumer relationship, to make a valuable contribution to the genetic decision process.

Some consumers have noted that their physician (whether their family doctor or a specialist) was not particularly helpful. Sometimes this was attributed to the physician's lack of familiarity with a rare disorder. Those living with the disorder felt that they were clearly more knowledgeable than the physician. More often, it was felt that the physician, though well informed in other matters, lacked sufficient knowledge of genetics or of the nature of DNA tests to provide help. Genetic counselors and other genetic professionals were, on the other hand, widely regarded as skilled in providing background and necessary interpretations, without being intrusive or judgmental. Frequently, it was the counselor/consumer relationship that was pivotal in easing the way to an informed decision. However, there were often practical impediments to this relationship, preventing it from becoming more central to the deliberations about DNA testing. Sometimes the genetic counseling clinic was located at a considerable distance. Even when it was not, the absence of a history of ongoing contact with the genetic professionals tended to place them in a peripheral position in the eyes of some of the consumers.

There is another valuable reservoir of expertise that has only recently begun to be tapped. It consists of those people who have already been through the demanding and draining process of making decisions about genetic testing. Consumers who have talked with such veterans, individuals who had, as one young father said, "walked in those same shoes," typically found much more than a receptive ear. They found people who were sensitive and sensible, who could raise issues without raising hackles, and who were generous in digging deep into their personal experience in order to share it with another. For the most part, such contacts came about through chance meetings at a clinic or a support group social event. Increasingly, lay organizations are becoming more active in helping to forge these contacts. Ways to reach organizations that are endeavoring to put people in touch with each other are discussed in Chapter Eight and listed in the Appendix.

Surprisingly, there is one group that is almost never consulted about genetic testing. This is so even though its representatives are well experienced in dealing with value-laden issues, are usually located conveniently close to home, and are dedicated to assisting people at critical junctures in their lives. That group is the clergy. Among the consumers I interviewed, many were deeply devoted to their own religious tradition and relied on their religious values as they made decisions about genetic testing. Yet very few consulted with their religious leader when decisions were being made. Part of the reason for this was doubt about the degree of genetic knowledge possessed by those with theological training. Sometimes it was a pastor's rigidity in making judgments, or the fact that the position of the religious group as a whole was well known and was perceived as unyielding, that led parishioners to conclude that there was little point in raising the issue. "You knew what the answer would be ahead of time," was a frequent comment. Some Catholics felt that celibate priests lacked understanding of family issues or a sensitivity to issues related to reproduction. The wall of silence shutting out the clergy tends to be breached only for very practical purposes, for example, when making arrangements with Sunday School teachers, or when trying to arrange wheelchair access for handicapped individuals into architecturally daunting church buildings.

Genetic problems, particularly when they affect children, have brought on crises of faith. One father likened himself to Ivan, in Dostoyevsky's *The Brothers Karamazov*, to explain why personally observing the suffering of his young child had a profound impact in turning him away from his former beliefs. "The dozens of times I had to hold down my child while doctors searched for a vein to take blood from does something to you. It makes you cold and cynical," said another parent. However, one woman found that her child's situation helped reinforce her religious identification. "I feel privileged and honored to have been given this child to raise."

Genetic counselors have noted instances when clergy have given good nondirective counseling. Increasingly, religious community representatives are trying to educate themselves in scientific and genetic matters so that they will have the background to enable them to deal with genetic issues. There are now some members of the clergy who work in the area of genetic counseling, and others who are even participating in clinical research. In the future, the clergy or its affiliated organizations may be more active in providing assistance to consumers facing genetic decisions.

Even while consumers have sought to consult with others whose input could be helpful, they have found it necessary to fend off *unwanted* advice. This advice often comes in the form of casual comments made by friends, baby-sitters, co-workers, and other outsiders who are pushing their own personal preferences. There are also widespread views that can influence people. They come from the broader social setting—in the unspoken messages deeply embedded in current medical custom and the steady drumbeat of messages from groups promoting social or religious agendas. On one side, there is the view that if a medical test is available, then it must be important and you are obliged to take it, as well as the view that a test somehow sets a standard and that you must pass it to have an acceptable "quality of life." On the other side, there is the view that one should never do anything to interfere with "nature" in any way. Consumers have been bombarded from both directions by these views. They have almost always found them irritating, intrusive, and distinctly unhelpful. Distancing oneself from them is not easy, but it is necessary.

Sample Decisions about Genetic Testing

In Chapter One, we met with several people, each of whom was faced with the fact that a serious health disorder brought about by a change in a single gene had suddenly appeared in their families. Let us return to see how the Stones, the MacFarlanes, and the Tates proceeded to gain answers to their questions and how, once it arose, they dealt with the opportunity to have genetic testing.

THE STONES' DECISION

Andrew and Donna Stone's little daughter, Melissa, was born with spinal muscular atrophy, SMA. Their concerns about how this had occurred in their family, and what their prospects were for having a child without genetic illness, had to be put on hold as they marshaled their resources (physical, emotional, and financial) to take care of their child. But whenever they could find islands of time, they tried to get information about SMA. They obtained medical articles from a friend who was a nurse. They began to have contact with an organization called National Families with SMA. From these sources, they learned that the gene for SMA had been localized to a spot on chromosome 5, and that there was a genetic test—a linkage test at that time—that could be used to track the gene.

They wanted more children and intended to have prenatal testing at the next pregnancy. Their biggest worry was not what having another affected child would do to them but "that the child would have to be put through so much." In speaking of their firstborn, they shared these thoughts: "Melissa was a special little girl—and she was happy. That was our biggest concern. The majority of the time when she wasn't being suctioned or filled with medications, she did lead a happy existence."

Shortly after Melissa died, Donna became pregnant again. Though they had planned to have prenatal testing, they had not made any advance preparations to see if their DNA markers were such that linkage testing would be possible. Why hadn't they checked into this before the pregnancy? Donna explained: "We wanted to keep Melissa at home. Caring for her was an around-the-clock obligation. From exhaustion, and then grief, we just weren't thinking clearly." Fortunately for the Stones, the laboratory quickly got back test results which showed that they had informative markers near the SMA gene. Those tests had required blood samples from both parents and also from Melissa, the individual with the disorder. A sample of Melissa's blood had been stored before her death. Without that stored sample, no linkage studies would have been possible.

The next step was the examination of the DNA from the fetal cells. This established that the fetus, a female, had a 99 percent chance of being free of SMA, though a carrier like her parents. A year after Kara's birth, they celebrated the birth of another healthy little girl (after again using DNA testing), this time a noncarrier.

During the whole process, the only time they had genetic counseling was prior to the chorionic villus sampling procedure used for collecting the cells needed for the prenatal DNA test. They had done most of the information gathering themselves. Melissa's pediatrician helped with the arrangements to draw and ship the blood samples to the commercial laboratory, where the actual DNA analysis was carried out. Paying for the genetic tests was a big problem, since medical expenses put them heavily in debt, but Andrew's brother helped out with a loan.

Donna's parents, who lived in another state, also provided blood samples, which were shipped separately to the laboratory. These additional samples were not required for the prenatal test, but her parents wanted to know which of them was a carrier and had passed the gene on to Donna. This would allow them to alert others on that side of the family to the possibility they could also be carriers. None of Donna's siblings has decided to determine their carrier status. Andrew's parents felt insulted when approached with the idea of including their samples with those being sent off to the laboratory, because they denied that the recessive gene could have come from either of them. (Of course, unless a very rare new mutation had occurred, one of them must have carried the gene.) It was only after Kara's birth that the normally warm relationship between Andrew and his parents was restored.

THE MACFARLANES' DECISION

For Harry and Jackie MacFarlane, hearing that their son Arthur had Duchenne muscular dystrophy was the beginning of a painful process of trying to find out on their own about his condition and about the possible risks to others in the family. Harry was very frustrated in his attempts to get information from the medical community and found that the material supplied by the Muscular Dystrophy Association was not detailed enough. He and his wife proceeded to get most of the information about the disorder from books and medical encyclopedias they found in their local library.

Arthur's DNA was tested, and the defect on his X chromosome was discovered. He was missing a small section of the gene that produces dystrophin, a muscle protein. The absence of normal dystrophin protein from muscle fibers accelerates the breakdown of muscles and will at some point require that Arthur get around with the aid of a wheelchair. The knowledge that the disorder is X-linked and that it is the dystrophin-forming gene that is involved means that Jackie MacFarlane would be able to have her own DNA tested. She could use a direct DNA test to find whether she is a carrier or whether Arthur has a new mutation (not unusual for this X-linked disorder). However, Jackie prefers not to know if she is a carrier. Based on what they have read, their opposition to abortion, and what they believe to be the best for their family, the MacFarlanes have decided not to have any more children. For them, testing Jackie's DNA is unnecessary since it will provide information that they neither want nor need.

Their other child, a daughter, has just turned ten. When she is older, perhaps in her midteens, and starting to think about her future family, they plan to tell her of the possibility that she may be a carrier. They will leave it up to her to make the decision about whether and when to have direct DNA testing. Jackie's sister, Jessie, could also be at risk. She is newly married and looking forward to having children, and the MacFarlanes have shared what they have learned with her. Jessie wants to have the testing done and will do so as soon as she and her husband have put aside enough money to pay for it. Others of Jackie's female relatives who may be at risk will be more difficult to contact. The family has never been close. Jackie is hoping that, little by little, word of her son's condition will work its way through this branch of the family and that others can mention this to their own physicians, especially when they become pregnant. The MacFarlanes are finding it easier to share what they know with others outside their own family circle. They are planning to start a support group in their region so that the search for information will not be so difficult for others as it has been for them.

THE TATES' DECISION

Karl Tate's parents never believed in going to doctors. As a child growing up in a rural community, the only time Karl saw the inside of a doctor's office was when he needed shots so that he could go to school or required stitches when there was an accident. His vision was not good, but he had never had his eyes tested for glasses until he went to work and could pay for them on his own. So it was no surprise to him, when his older brother was diagnosed with neurofibromatosis (NF1), that his parents denied any possibility that the disease could have been inherited and they buried the information. The many skin discolorations (called cafe-au-lait spots) that can be an indicator of NF1, and the small tumors which they all saw on his father's body when he rested out in the backyard in warm weather, were dismissed by his mother as "beauty marks."

Still, Karl was terribly unhappy that no word of his brother's condition was communicated to him. And his wife Phyllis was in a panic and furious that neither his parents nor his brother thought to contact others in the family. As soon as they returned home from the wedding where they first got the news about Karl's brother, Karl and Phyllis went to their internist to find out more about NF1. The doctor thought that Karl showed no signs of it and, because he was already in his thirties, was almost certainly unaffected. The doctor was less sure about the availability of genetic testing, but did refer them to a genetic counseling unit at a nearby medical center. The counselor there was able to explain the dominant pattern of inheritance of NF1 and the details of the linkage test that can track the gene in families. Should they wish to proceed with genetic studies, a blood sample from Karl's father would have to be obtained.

A number of factors combined to influence their decision not to have genetic testing. They were reassured by the fact that Karl showed no signs of NF1, and that the symptoms in the members of the Tate family known to have the disorder were fairly mild. Even if they had tried to force the issue, it was most unlikely that Karl's father would have agreed to have his blood drawn for the linkage test. And there was a small risk that obtaining fetal cells for a prenatal test could cause a spontaneous abortion.

Their genetic counseling experience was a very good one and they were grateful for the information and the explanations that the counselor was able to provide. Less successful was their attempt to locate other families with the disorder so that they could benefit from their experience. A phone message left at the number of a neuro-fibromatosis support group went unreturned. Also surprising was their discovery that, had they decided to proceed with the DNA test, they would have had to pay all the bills themselves. According to the terms of their health plan, the insurance company would reimburse them for the costs of testing of a possibly affected child, but would not pay for testing a fetus.

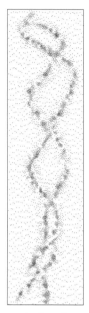

Chapter Five

Making Decisions about Testing for Susceptibility

S ophie Baldwin glows with good health. She takes care to eat a nutritious diet. She runs two miles each day along the beaches near her home and gets plenty of rest each night. Yet Sophie fears that, like her mother and most of the other women in her family, she will die young—from breast cancer.

Many of us know of the diseases that afflicted our grandparents and parents. We vaguely suspect that the same diseases might be lying in wait for us as well. Up until recently, there has been little understanding of how common illnesses like cancer, heart disease, diabetes, or Alzheimer's disease seemed to run in families. For the most part, these illnesses are not like the single-gene disorders that were the focus of Chapter Four. For single-gene disorders, we were able to refer to well-established rules of inheritance (dominant, recessive, X-linked) to explain their occurrence. But for many common health problems, the patterns of inheritance are far more complicated.

These types of illnesses are known as "multifactorial" or "complex" disorders. They involve many external contributing elements—including diet, lifestyle, exposure to drugs, chemicals, or infections—that interact in complicated ways with elements within our body, such as our genes. Except in rare cases, genes by themselves do not determine the outcome. However, scientists have begun to appreciate that the presence of certain genes may change the odds of developing an illness. Like the butcher's thumb pressed on the weighing pan, certain versions of genes tip the scales so that a person is predisposed to develop particular problems. We have always to keep in mind, however, that though genes may play a role, they are only some of the actors among a whole cast of environmental characters that need to be assembled before a disease actually occurs.

Cancer, heart disease, Alzheimer's disease, and diabetes are among our major health problems. They take a huge personal and societal toll. Much recent scientific research has been focused on finding out more about how these problems occur. The goal of this research is to come up with better ways of treating these disorders when they do occur and better ways of preventing them. As a result, genetic and nongenetic contributions to these problems are being sought and some have been identified.

In this chapter we will look at genetic testing that can provide information about susceptibility to disorders. We are witnessing the earliest stages of this new category of genetic testing, and our experience with it is still limited. We will see that the same four factors that are central to decision making for the single-gene disorders discussed in Chapter Four apply here as well. That is, before going on with testing, one should consider (1) the features of the disorder; (2) the requirements of the test; (3) the timing of the testing; and (4) the options or opportunities that testing unlocks as well as those that it blocks. However, several features of susceptibility testing may cause consumers to weigh these factors somewhat differently than they would for single-gene disorders, as they make decisions about genetic testing.

Identifying Genes Associated with Susceptibility

When different elements jointly contribute to the onset of a disease, then determining the importance of any individual one is a difficult process. First of all, not every disorder has a genetic basis. Scientists must find out whether genes are significantly involved at all. If genes are involved, then identifying which ones they are is a laborious task.

In doing research to identify genes that predispose a person to a disorder, scientists start by studying a few families in which there happen to be a large number of cases of the same disorder. The occurrence of an unusually large cluster of cases within a family (at least two or more affected individuals who are closely related to each other) can be a sign of a genetic component. Another clue is that the first symptoms appear at a younger age in this family than in most people with the disorder. Breast cancer diagnosed in young women in their twenties or thirties (rather than in old age) is such a clue. Still another signal indicating the involvement of genes is the occurrence of a disorder in both of the paired organs—in both breasts, or both eyes, or both kidneys. Having a problem occur very early, or occur twice in the same individual, seems to indicate that more than random events are taking place and that genes may be setting the stage for an illness.

The incidence of a disease for identical twins, when compared to the incidence for fraternal twins, is another way to see how much of a contribution can be assigned to genes. Twins growing up at the same time and in the same place share pretty much the same environment. Where they can differ is in the number of genes they share. Identical twins, resulting as they do from the same fertilized egg, have all the same genes. Fraternal twins, resulting from the fertilization of two different eggs by different sperm, have half their genes in common (as would any two siblings). If both members of sets of identical twins are found to develop a disorder more frequently than both members of sets of fraternal twins, the conclusion is drawn that some of the genes shared by the identical twins must be important in triggering the disorder.

Once the evidence pointing to a genetic component begins to accumulate, gene searching tools can be pressed into service. An assortment of DNA markers is used to get a fix on where the actual genes reside on the chromosomes. If the same marker appears to be present in all the affected family members, then a variety of techniques can be used to close in on the gene. More than once, scientists thought they had "captured" a potential susceptibility gene, only to discover, on more careful analysis, that they could find no changes or mutations in that gene in individuals having the disorder. Thus, even when a likely gene candidate is found, it is necessary to show that individuals who have the disorder have changes or mutations in that gene that do not occur in individuals who do not have the disorder. Once a gene has been identified and the specific (illness-causing) changes in the DNA are known, it becomes possible to develop tests to look for those mutations in other family members, as yet unaffected, or in other families where the disorder has already appeared. The cluster of cases of early-onset breast cancer marks Sophie Baldwin's family as one in which genes may be present that predispose its members to breast cancer.

A Few Notes of Caution

Not every cluster of cases of a disorder in a family can be taken as a sure sign that susceptibility genes are involved. The kinds of disorders we are talking about here are all very common indeed. They are disorders that are so prevalent that they have assumed the status of major public health problems. Because they are so common it can happen that, by chance alone, several family members can have the very same disorder. For example, about one woman in nine will develop breast cancer during her lifetime, if she lives into her eighties. Therefore, the occurrence of extended families in which two or three or even more women have developed breast cancer is not unusual. In fact, it is *expected* to happen in some (unlucky) families purely on probability grounds alone, in the complete absence of any genes that predispose to that illness. The same is true for heart disease, Alzheimer's disease, or any other common disease.

Not every research report holds up. Looking for markers that can help pinpoint the genes that make us more susceptible to a disorder is a very difficult and tricky task. An early report that tentatively locates a gene at one spot on a chromosome is often overturned after more information is collected. In a study of a large family, researchers thought they had identified on chromosome 11 a DNA marker close to a gene for bipolar disorder. But it turned out to be a false lead after two family members *without* the marker were later found to have the disorder. Chromosome regions once thought to harbor susceptibility genes have later been exonerated after more data were gathered. It is wise for consumers to remain cautious, particularly of accounts found in the popular media, and to wait until the necessary confirming studies are concluded. Confirming the identity of a susceptibility gene is, scientifically, a hard problem that takes time.

Not every variation occurring in the DNA of a gene leads to a major health problem down the line. Some variations are more meaningful than others. As we have seen in Chapter Two, there are many small variations in the DNA sequence scattered throughout our chromosomes. Some variations within a gene can occur without having any effect on the final protein product. Others may have a minimal or very mild effect. And some mutations change the properties of that protein product in ways that can have serious impact on one's present or future health. Until there is enough experience to be sure whether a particular change in the DNA leads to disease, it will be very hard to distinguish those DNA variations which cause a gene to trigger a health problem from those DNA variations which are innocuous, and do no harm.

Some Known Susceptibility Genes

Many different genes can predispose us to different types of health problems. Over time, as research proceeds, more of these genes will be identified. Right now, the number of susceptibility genes for which testing exists is small, but it is growing at a steady pace. Some of the first susceptibility genes found have been for breast cancer, colon cancer, and Alzheimer's disease. Here are a few examples.

CANCER SUSCEPTIBILITY

One cancer susceptibility gene, MSH2, is associated with colon cancer. The lifetime risk for developing the disease is 10 percent in the general population. But for the one in two hundred men and women who have inherited a flawed MSH2 gene, the chance of getting colon cancer is much higher, about 80 percent. Another susceptibility gene is called BRCA1 (for breast cancer 1). Mutant forms of BRCA1 increase the possibility a woman could develop breast cancer. From health statistics gathered in the United States, a woman has, on average, a one-in-nine or an 11 percent chance of developing breast cancer over her entire lifetime. It is estimated that about one in three hundred women have inherited one copy of a mutant BRCA1 gene. Women with this mutant gene have a probability of getting breast cancer that is much higher than 11 percent. Their chance of getting breast cancer by age fifty is 59 percent. If they live to age ninety, their chance of developing cancer by that age is 85 percent. They also have a much higher rate of ovarian cancer than women in the general population.

Cancer begins when a single cell, anywhere in the body, loses its ability to carefully control the way it divides. There are several steps that any healthy dividing cell needs to carry out. Division is such an important event that cells have several different genes which back each other up at each step. First of all, a cell must ensure that its DNA is accurately copied. MSH2 is one of a group of genes that function to repair errors in chromosomal DNA stemming from the occasional failure of the A, T, G, and C bases to form the proper A-T and G-C pairs when DNA is doubling. After chromosome doubling is completed, a healthy cell must keep the cell division process moving in an orderly manner by stimulating certain functions and suppressing others. BRCA1 is one of the genes which acts as a suppressor, keeping cell division from taking place too frequently, too quickly, or in an unrestrained fashion.

If one cell happens to contain about four to six mutated and impaired genes among those that regulate some aspect of the division process, that cell's control of division is irretrievably damaged. The cell can now divide wildly, producing a large mass of cells—or tumor—which has the potential to cause damage wherever it occurs. The tumor may go on to shed cells which spread around the body and take hold in other places, with life-threatening results.

How do mutations occur in otherwise functioning genes? Over time, our genes can suffer injury from the effects of agents that come from the outside environment: substances in air, water, and food; radiation; cigarette smoke; germs; and pollutants. More assaults on our DNA come from substances produced within our own bodies. There are by-products of the cell's normal chemical activities that are capable of damaging the cell's own genetic material. Our cells try to fix much of this damage, but the repair machinery is not perfect. On rare occasions, errors slip through and permanent mutations result. These are called *somatic mutations.* They can occur anytime during the course of our lives. These mutations can occur in cells of the liver, the lung, the pancreas, the prostate—in any part of our body. Given enough time, it can happen that one unfortunate cell acquires mutations in enough of the genes concerned with cell division to put an end to normal cell division. It usually takes a long time for that one unfortunate cell to accumulate the several different mutations that cause it to be the start of a tumor. It is for this reason that cancer is usually a disease of old age.

Susceptibility genes shorten the path for tumor formation. Suppose that a person has, through the egg or sperm, *inherited* a gene (like a mutated copy of the BRCA1 gene) that is unable to carry out one of the steps necessary for controlling cell division. If that has happened, then every cell in the body will have that particular damaged gene. This puts each cell in the unenviable position of being one step closer to becoming a cancer cell. It means that it takes fewer additional mutations to change a normal cell to a cancer cell. Thus the risk of developing cancer is higher for those with an inherited mutation than for those without such a mutation.

The BRCA1 gene is one example of a group of susceptibility genes called *tumor suppressors.* Tumor-suppressor genes act to quash the tendency of the cell to divide before it is ready. Inheriting one defective BRCA1 gene does not, by itself, cause a problem. It is like trying to pull on the reins of a galloping horse with one hand tied behind your back. It may be a little awkward to exert control, but it can be done. What would happen to a person who has inherited one flawed BRCA1 gene if the second BRCA1 gene should eventually become damaged and a mutation result? It would be like having both hands tied. Then it becomes impossible to use the reins to control the galloping horse. With no functional BRCA1 gene available, one important step in regulating the division process is now gone. In combination with other mutations that occur, over time, to a few other genes, the cell can now start to divide recklessly.

ALZHEIMER'S DISEASE SUSCEPTIBILITY

The accelerated death of brain cells, causing loss of memory and loss of the ability to function independently, are among the grim hallmarks of Alzheimer's disease. There is a rare early-onset form of this disease that is caused by inheriting a specific mutant gene (actually, any one of three such genes). This form, which appears before age sixty-five, is inherited as a single-gene disorder, like those discussed in Chapter Four. This early-onset form of Alzheimer's will not be discussed in this section.

The typical form of Alzheimer's disease is a late-onset disease. One gene that is prominently associated with the late-onset form is called the apolipoprotein E gene (apo-E for short). There are three variations of the apo-E gene. One of these, $\varepsilon 4$, is known to predispose to Alzheimer's disease. For individuals with no $\varepsilon 4$ gene, the risk of developing Alzheimer's disease by age eighty is about 20 percent. Individuals with just one copy of the $\varepsilon 4$ gene (estimated to be about 40 percent of the population) have about a 45 percent chance of developing the disease. Individuals who have inherited two $\varepsilon 4$ genes have a 90 percent chance of developing the disease. The genetic predisposition associated with the $\varepsilon 4$ gene is thus quite substantial. Still, it should be clear that the predisposition associated with the $\varepsilon 4$ gene does not represent a certainty of getting the disease. And the absence of $\varepsilon 4$ does not represent immunity from the disease. Alzheimer's disease occurs after a lifetime of exposure to all kinds of environmental influences such as diet, the occurrence of blows to the head, and exposure to toxins or infections. Genetics is just one part of the story.

The genetic roots of disorders that arise later in life (such as Alzheimer's disease and perhaps other major health problems as well) are already present at conception. Such disorders can be traced to small variations present in the DNA sequence of one or more genes. These DNA variations do not deliver a knockout punch, preventing the gene (or genes) from functioning. They probably bring about small changes in the way the gene carries out its function in the cell. The *amount* of protein the gene produces may be changed; for example, less than usual may be produced. Or the *properties* of the protein produced may be changed in subtle ways: The protein may work at a slightly different rate, making a chemical reaction in the cell occur faster or slower, or it may be a little less efficient in the way it coordinates with other proteins. In addition, the changed way that the gene functions may make the individual's health more vulnerable to environmental influences. If the protein's job is to neutralize a toxin that enters from the environment and if the protein produced by the altered gene is less effective at that job, then that toxin may do some damage.

Just as a tiny amount of water dripping steadily and over a long time can wear a hole in the surface of a rock, so a small change in the functioning of a gene (like the ε4 variation of the apo-E gene connected with Alzheimer's), acting steadily and over a long time, can damage an organ such as the brain. A gradual decline in the organ's vital processes may eventually result in a serious disorder.

SUSCEPTIBILITY TO OTHER HEALTH PROBLEMS

The tools of genetic analysis are now being pressed into service to help gain an understanding of other forms of cancer, as well as many other conditions that create substantial and often life-threatening problems for those affected. These include heart disease, diabetes, neurological disorders, and mental illness. Because it is the number one cause of death in Western countries, coronary artery disease has been at the center of attention for many researchers. Coronary artery disease occurs when fatty materials are deposited on the walls of blood vessels that nourish the heart, diminishing the blood supply to the heart and impairing heart function. If the heart's blood vessels become completely blocked, then a heart attack results. The search for a susceptibility gene is focusing on genes that are responsible for how fatty materials are transported through the blood and removed from it, genes that affect the clotting properties of blood, and genes that work to repair artery walls where fatty material settles. Several genes involved in these activities are strong candidates warranting further study.

Genes that predispose to other illnesses are also being sought. Families with a history of multiple cases of a disorder are being looked at in research studies. Researchers have identified some of those which are associated with juvenile diabetes (insulin dependent) as well as the adult (non-insulin dependent) type. Studies of asthma, rheumatoid arthritis, and multiple sclerosis are also pointing out possible predisposing genes. Among behavioral disorders, susceptibility genes have been implicated in schizophrenia, bipolar disorder, and alcohol abuse. Separating environmental from genetic factors for behavioral disorders is difficult. It is even harder than for physical illness. This makes the search for genes predisposing to behavioral disorders an especially unwieldy task, which can raise a lot of false leads.

Genetic Testing for Predisposition to Health Disorders

As more susceptibility genes are ferreted out of our total bank of genes, scientists will need to determine which alterations of these genes are associated with increased risk of illness and which are not. With that knowledge, DNA tests for those genes will be possible. Testing is already occurring, in commercial laboratories, for breast cancer and Alzheimer's disease susceptibility. Once again, consumers are faced with questions about whether they wish to have such tests done. Sophie Baldwin is one of those considering whether she should be tested to see if she has a mutant BRCA1 gene that would predispose her to breast cancer.

Our experience with genetic tests for determining susceptibility to disorders is limited. Very few genes have been identified. Existing tests are quite new. Most people who have already had the tests have done so while enrolled as research subjects in pilot studies for breast cancer susceptibility. Still, it is possible to describe the factors that are pertinent to decisions about this type of genetic testing. One can look closely at the reports of these early studies and then consider them in light of the experiences of those who, in the absence of testing, are anxiously considering how to deal with what they see as a dark cloud of disease hanging over their family.

Using these data, it appears that the same four factors that figure so importantly in decisions about testing for single-gene disorders also apply to decisions about genetic testing for susceptibility.

The Disorder

As with the single-gene disorders, the kinds of health problems that could result from having a susceptibility gene, as well as the available treatments, are fundamental to any decision making about testing. Cancer, heart disease, diabetes, and most of the health problems at issue here, occur so frequently that the degree of our familiarity with them can be substantial. These illnesses are the subject of books and movies. Information about them is featured in news reports. They are brought to our homes by neighbors collecting funds for national organizations like the American Cancer Society or the American Heart Association. The willingness of people in the public eye to share details of their personal experiences also contributes to greater awareness. Betty Ford's openness about having breast cancer and Ronald Reagan's disclosure that he was diagnosed to have Alzheimer's disease are two of many examples.

In addition to this general background of information, there may also be a lot of direct personal knowledge. The disorders associated with an inherited susceptibility gene can appear in every generation as the gene is passed from parent to child. In some families, where the illness has appeared frequently, it can have the appearance of a dominant pattern of inheritance. Having affected relatives provides powerful lessons. For Sophie Baldwin, watching her mother battle breast cancer was her main source of education. Memories of her mother being "hacked to bits and filled with chemicals and radiation" are etched in her mind. Even though she was seventeen years old when her mother died, these memories—and the feelings they engendered—continue to mold her current view about the burden of breast cancer. For other women, there has been a different take-home lesson: Seeing family members alive and well twenty years after being diagnosed as having cancer makes the burden seem less heavy and little different from other disorders that can be managed, and even defeated, with current treatments.

The Test

The genetic tests employed to detect susceptibility genes usually (but not always) are direct tests. Testing DNA for a gene that predisposes to future illness comes with its own share of difficulties at the beginning, before the test is even conducted. This type of testing also carries its own uncertainties, once a result has been obtained. Both of these aspects of the testing process figure prominently in whether consumers choose to proceed with susceptibility testing.

GATHERING FAMILY INFORMATION

Accurate knowledge of one's family history is an important prerequisite for susceptibility gene testing. The health problems experienced by older family members may herald the kinds of health problems that younger members of the family may face. Layers of confusion may need to be penetrated before the real family medical history becomes clear and a pattern emerges that points to the possible involvement of a susceptibility gene.

Studies have shown that the information we possess about first-degree relatives (parents and siblings) is generally quite reliable, especially if the disease caused someone to die. But for chronic diseases that did not cause death, and for more distant relations like aunts, uncles, and grandparents, information about medical problems may not be reliable at all. The embarrassment and dread that in the past has been associated with many illnesses like Alzheimer's disease and cancer meant that they tended to be spoken of only in hushed tones, if they were mentioned at all. When death occurred, the cause was often shrouded in mystery: The only explanation given was that death came "after a long illness." Sometimes, the diagnosis given to explain observed symptoms turned out to be incorrect. For example, adverse reactions to drugs sometimes produce symptoms that mimic those of a chronic disorder. This has sometimes misled family members and medical professionals into thinking that Alzheimer's disease or mental illness was present when, in fact, it was not.

It may be possible to obtain medical records to reconstruct an accurate health history. But this is often hard. One must first find out where records are kept. Knowing the name of the doctor who treated the individual or the hospital in which a person died is essential. Keep in mind that many institutions hold on to medical records only for seven to ten years before discarding them. Gaining access to someone else's private records requires permission. Some documents (such as death certificates) may turn out to be incomplete. It will take perseverance, time, and more than a little luck to collect the relevant information. In the absence of such data, personal records, like the items recorded in some family bibles, may be useful in assessing whether genetic predispositions exist. Medical professionals and national health organizations encourage people to start their own family health history, with names of doctors and hospitals listed, and to update it on a regular basis.

Medical geneticists are still just beginning to learn which versions of a gene may predispose to illness, and which do not or do so only rarely. As progress is made in uncovering the genetic component of a common illness, they will more clearly identify those mutations that are definitely connected with increased risk for that illness. If there has been any previous genetic testing of members of the family affected with the disorder, it is extremely helpful to know the results of those tests. When a particular susceptibility gene mutation—or DNA marker for that gene—is found in the family, future testing of as-yet-unaffected family members can focus on that specific genetic alteration or DNA marker. In the absence of a known mutation or marker specific to the family, it may not be practical or financially possible to test a person for all mutations connected with increased risk.

Having access to stored tissue or tumor samples may make it possible to look for the presence of a susceptibility gene with DNA tests that only became available after that person's death. Stored tissue is critical if linkage testing is being considered in families where the affected members have died.

INTERPRETING TEST RESULTS

When we considered DNA linkage tests in Chapter Four, we saw that there was an uncertainty that accompanied the test results. After all, a linkage test cannot tell for sure whether the nearby target gene— the gene that will bring on a disorder—is actually present. The test can only predict the chance, or probability, that the target gene was inherited. Many consumers feel that linkage tests must provide a high predicted probability (greater than 90 percent) before they are worth doing. The lower the predicted probability a test could provide (for the presence of the target gene), the less willing people are to undergo the test.

Uncertainty also appears in drawing conclusions from test results when the target is a susceptibility gene. But the uncertainty here is of a different sort. A direct DNA test will be able to establish whether the version of a gene that predisposes to the illness is present. But finding that a single susceptibility gene is present does not mean that the corresponding illness will ever develop. This additional uncertainty is tied to the fact that the susceptibility gene is just one component among a number of genetic and environmental components that together can combine to bring on the illness. Fifteen percent of women born with a mutant BRCA1 gene will never develop breast or ovarian cancer in their lifetime. Fifty-five percent of those born with an ε4 gene have no signs of Alzheimer's disease at age eighty. Thus a factor to consider when deciding whether to test is the probability of escaping the illness, even if test results reveal the presence of a susceptibility gene.

By the same token, because these disorders occur even in the absence of the susceptibility gene, a finding that the gene is absent is no guarantee someone will be spared. The large majority of breast cancer cases occur in women who have no detectable susceptibility gene. Heart disease and diabetes occur to those with none of the known susceptibility genes. So, this is another factor to consider: the probability of developing the illness even if test results indicate the absence of a susceptibility gene. Decisions about testing will also be tied to costs of the DNA tests compared to the costs of others that can pick up predisposing symptoms (such as blood pressure measurements for cardiac problems, blood tests of stool samples for colon cancer).

The Timing

For most of the disorders where predisposing genes are present, the first symptoms appear in the adult years. This means that there can be a long time delay between when a test reveals the presence of a susceptibility gene and when the first symptoms of a health problem appear. Perhaps because people have many productive years before the onset of problems (or because they recognize that, as theologian J. Robert Nelson put it, we are *all* born with a disease called "mortality" which will come upon us in ways we cannot anticipate) there has been little interest thus far in pursuing prenatal testing for these disorders. Although families who learn during pregnancy of a potential risk for their children often feel great urgency about testing, urgency is seldom present when susceptibility testing is involved. Consumers do not have the need to keep one eye on a rapidly ticking clock. There will be adequate time to go ahead with testing later, if they wish to do so.

Stage-of-life issues do arise with susceptibility testing. Is it appropriate to use these tests to find out the genetic status of children? Should a young girl be tested for the BRCA1 mutation that will predispose her to breast cancer? Does it make sense to look for susceptibility to heart disease in a teenage boy? The answers to such questions are no more settled here than they were for single-gene disorders.

Most guidelines put forth by professional groups support the testing of children only when there is a real medical benefit possible for the child. Such a benefit exists when there is some way to counteract the action of a susceptibility gene and avoid the potential illness. Alternatively, testing that shows that the mutant gene was not inherited would spare a child the unpleasant diagnostic tests that are used to catch some illnesses in their early stages. If the information gained from the test would not accomplish either goal, then the potential for inflicting emotional harm, should the test show an increased risk (and mark the child as different from other siblings), would make testing unacceptable.

Some genetic professionals believe that there are occasions, admittedly rare ones, that justify giving these tests to children. For some children, the fear of getting the same life-threatening illness that has stricken a parent is an ever-present part of their lives. This fear may color the way they think about themselves and could sabotage their hopes for the future. Pre-adolescent girls have been seen pounding on their breasts, trying to keep them from growing, so that they wouldn't have to suffer like their mothers. If they were tested, half of these girls would be found not to have the family susceptibility gene for breast cancer; these children could be reassured and released from anxiety. The other half, found to have the gene, could be encouraged to begin making beneficial risk-reducing changes in diet and lifestyle. These changes would be more effective in lowering risk than similar changes begun later on in life. Thus, there are circumstances in which a consideration of the likely benefits and harms would make susceptibility testing of children an appropriate step. As with any type of medical intervention, it is the well-being of the child—not the anxieties and concerns felt by the parents or by anyone else—that must be paramount.

The Options

One key characteristic that distinguishes susceptibility testing from other types of genetic testing (such as the presymptomatic testing discussed in Chapter Four) are the new options that it provides. Those found to have a susceptibility gene can take two types of action that may substantially reduce their chances of contracting the illness:

- Modify patterns of diet, exercise, smoking, and other lifestyle habits. Studies show that these changes are effective in reducing the incidence of many chronic diseases.
- Put in place a program of careful medical surveillance. Depending on the disorder for which one is at risk, this might include

mammograms, colonoscopies, blood tests, and cardiograms. (There is a special genetic circumstance when mammography may not be recommended. This is discussed at the end of this section on options, on page 122.) Regular health monitoring may enable a person to pick up the first warning signs of impending problems, possibly in time to reverse them. If treatments are available, they could be started at an early stage of an illness when they usually work best.

Of course, one does not have to be tested and shown to have a susceptibility gene before taking these two types of actions. For years, doctors have been advising their patients to follow both courses of action as a matter of prudent health practice. And many people, just on the basis of their family history, have been motivated to follow this advice. Finding out that you actually do have a susceptibility gene may provide an even stronger incentive.

Some people at risk for cancer have an additional option. They can undergo "prophylactic" (preventive) surgery to remove the healthy organ in which a malignant cell is most likely to arise. This medical procedure—called prophylactic mastectomy (when the breasts are removed) or prophylactic oophorectomy (when the ovaries are removed)—is taken to eliminate the most vulnerable tissues before a malignancy starts. Prophylactic surgery has been proven to work in familial polyposis coli and in multiple endocrine neoplasia 2A (MEN2A). These are two rare forms of cancer in which inherited mutations in a single gene seem to initiate an inevitable progression to early colon cancer or thyroid cancer. For these disorders, the surgical removal of the colon or the thyroid gland is usually curative.

For breast cancer, even before any susceptibility genes were identified, there were women who opted for prophylactic surgery because of a family history of this illness. Fearful that they were at high risk, they saw it as a way to reduce their chance of breast cancer or of ovarian cancer. One woman, an oncology nurse, preferred the surgery because of her observations of what some patients had to endure in regimens of chemotherapy used after cancer develops. Another woman selected prophylactic surgery because she wanted to be as sure as she could be that she would see her young children grow up. For her, the surgery seemed to be the best way to accomplish this. It has allowed her to feel good about herself and relieved her of the anxiety that she had felt on a daily basis.

In families where a dominant susceptibility gene is being passed on, each family member has an equal chance of inheriting that gene or of being spared the gene. In the past, many women chose prophylactic surgery without knowing their genetic status. Through the use of a genetic test, *only* those who are found to have the gene (and who are indeed at higher risk) may wish to consider it.

Prophylactic surgery is a difficult option. It is a major and invasive procedure. Removal of the breasts entails loss of the nipples and all the associated tissue, leading to a loss of sensation. Removal of the ovaries, especially after a woman has completed her family, may be an easier decision to make. The ovaries are not visible and their hormones can be supplied in the form of pills. What is not certain is whether either type of surgery is completely effective. Since breast tissue is not as well defined as, for example, colon or thyroid tissue, it is possible that some remnants may be left behind that could become the starting point of a malignancy. There have been reports of women who underwent ovary removal only to have a cancer cell form on the adjacent tissue in the lining of the abdominal cavity. Studies are needed to examine the incidence of cancer in women who have had this surgery and to establish reliably just how protective it really is. At present, prophylactic surgery is not covered in many health insurance plans.

Information about genetic susceptibility can encourage consumers to take action that could reduce their risk and improve their prospects for a healthier future. That same information carries with it what is perhaps the biggest problem associated with susceptibility testing. It is possible that information about a genetic predisposition to a chronic, costly, and sometimes incapacitating condition could be used by others as the justification for denying consumers access to insurance coverage, job opportunities, or admittance into educational programs.

Use (and misuse) of genetic information by others is a problem that was discussed in Chapter Four in connection with single-gene disorders, and it will be discussed in more detail in Chapter Six. It is a serious consideration for susceptibility testing. Most of the disorders for which susceptibility tests are being carried out are the very disorders that are customarily used to evaluate one's likely future health status. This type of genetic information would surely be of interest in setting rates for health or life insurance, judging a prospective employee's ability to do a job, or choosing which among many deserving candidates should be selected when there are a limited number of slots in an educational or training program.

Many consumers, concerned about how this genetic information might be used, have paid for the tests themselves so their health insurance companies would not know anything about it. They have sought to keep test results out of their medical records. The possibility that personal genetic information may be misused or unfairly used must be included in any decision about undergoing susceptibility testing.

The sharing of test results *within the family* raises other issues that are similar to those for single-gene disorders. Revealing one's own results to others will compromise privacy. It could lead to survivor guilt among those family members who learn that they have not inherited the susceptibility gene. At the same time, knowing that there is a genetic predisposition in the family may help foster wiser decisions about health habits and will allow relatives to make their own choices about DNA testing. In some ways, the information-sharing issues are moderated by the fact that, in contrast to the single-gene situation, a susceptibility gene is only one among many components that contribute to a disorder. It's quite possible that family members have already learned of their potential risk. Their own doctors should pick up on this when they take a family history.

A Special Circumstance in Breast Cancer

Regular mammography screening is the centerpiece of most breast cancer surveillance programs. A mammogram is a photograph taken with X-rays instead of visible light. Mammograms enable cancer within the breast to be spotted when still very small and localized and most treatable.

There is one unusual situation when such screening has the potential for being more harmful than helpful. There is a rare single-gene disorder called ataxia telangiectasia. Affected children who have inherited two flawed recessive genes, one from each carrier parent, suffer from a number of serious problems. These include balance problems, immune system impairment, extreme sensitivity to radiation, and in some cases the development of cancers of the blood. The specific gene involved (named ATM) plays a critical role in the repair of any damage inflicted on DNA by radiation. Mutations in this gene permit the cell to go ahead and divide before it has finished making repairs to its DNA. This means that some damage caused by radiation does not get repaired and becomes fixed in the DNA as a permanent mutation.

Studies have shown that carriers of the ATM gene, who are estimated at about 1 percent of the population, have a fourfold higher risk for all types of cancer. Women who are carriers have a fivefold higher risk for breast cancer.

Mammography involves small amounts of X-ray exposure. Since carriers of the ATM gene may be more sensitive to radiation, there is a real possibility that, for such carriers, the very procedure used for detecting malignancies may itself contribute to the future appearance of a malignant cell. Women who are found to be carriers of this gene would want to consider other kinds of surveillance strategies.

Making a Decision about Susceptibility Testing

Just as we have noted in Chapter Four, consumers considering genetic testing have found that four factors (the disorder, the test, the timing, and the options) should be evaluated separately and then in combination with each other, when coming to a decision. Part of this decision process requires knowing what medical monitoring can be done and what demands and costs this type of ongoing surveillance would entail. It would require knowing what kinds of lifestyle changes or medications could help prevent a disorder and what, if anything, could be done to deal with it if it appears. To gain this type of information means that there is a need to consult closely with health-care providers. The physician/patient relationship, with its traditional emphasis on the well-being of the patient, remains as pivotal for susceptibility testing as it is for other types of genetic testing. Here too, having the opportunity to benefit from the experiences of other people who have faced these very same concerns can provide consumers with additional sources of insight and a sympathetic sounding board as decisions are being made. Ways of contacting and consulting others who have been in the same boat are presented in Chapter Eight and outlined in the Appendix.

SOPHIE BALDWIN'S DECISION

Sophie Baldwin found out about genetic testing from a health magazine. At first, the possibility that she could have genetic testing seemed like a dream come true. A few years ago, she had given very serious thought to having a prophylactic mastectomy, but summed up her decision against it with the comment: "I'm attached to my boobs." Now, with the prospect of a DNA test, she looked forward to finally knowing if her chances of getting breast cancer were high—or if she was at no greater risk than any other woman in the general population. "If I find out that I haven't inherited the gene, I'll go back to school and figure out how to live forty more years, planning for menopause and old age."

Since all her relatives with breast cancer are now deceased and, as far as Sophie knows, no blood or tissue taken from her mother was ever stored, there would be no way to know whether her mother or any of her relatives had a particular BRCA1 mutation. Her gynecologist explained it would be possible to send a sample of her own blood to a commercial laboratory that specializes in this type of testing. There, they could test for several of the most common mutations in the BRCA1 gene. If the laboratory did not find any of these common mutations, it still would not rule out that another BRCA1 mutation—not searched for in the test—was present. And it would not preclude there being another, completely different gene that, in her family, brought with it the high risk for breast cancer.

At first Sophie was eager to go ahead with the testing. But then she began to wonder who else would get their hands on this information.

She was insured through her employer in a group plan. What would happen if she ever left for another job and had to apply to a new health plan? Would she have to reveal the test results? Could this become a "pre-existing condition" that would make her uninsurable? Until she knew the answers to these questions, she reluctantly put aside her plans for genetic testing. Her fear of having the test results used against her more than matched her fear of cancer.

So Sophie continues to follow as healthy a lifestyle as she can, to do monthly self-exams of her breasts, and to have an annual mammogram. She has elected to wait to see what laws or policies may be put in place that might spare her what she views as the double jeopardy of a genetic test: finding out she has a susceptibility gene and then discovering that the health care she will need to find and treat breast cancer early, when chances of a cure are highest, will be denied to her.

Trends

The DNA susceptibility tests now available are in the vanguard of tests that can identify the diseases that we are likely to be locked in battle with in the years to come. Already there is talk of going beyond testing those in families with a history of a disease to testing the general population routinely—much as cholesterol screening or blood-pressure screening are used today.

Such proposals are premature. We are only in the early stages of this form of testing. Much remains to be learned scientifically. The correlation between a specific mutation in a gene and its ultimate impact on the health of an individual is known only for those families in which the mutation produces a definite effect on health. Studies must be done to ascertain which genetic changes are meaningful and which are not. The mechanisms by which any of these genes and environmental factors interact to produce illness are still unknown. We must also learn how to explain what these tests mean so that people are not unduly alarmed or falsely reassured.

Finally, there is much that we need to learn about the consequences to individuals should others obtain this kind of information about them. We need to develop ways of protecting people who are found to possess susceptibility genes from stigmatization and from discrimination. In Chapter Six, we will look at the current laws and regulations with respect to revealing genetic test results, and we will look at the policies being proposed to help shield consumers from harm. Until good policies are established, susceptibility tests should be used with care—and only by individuals whose family histories indicate that genes that predispose them to illness may be present.

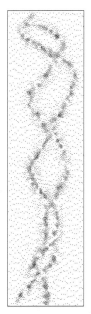

Chapter Six

Societal Uses of DNA Testing Information

G enetics is not just a personal and family matter. Genetic information has long been of interest to outsiders. This interest has sometimes had unfortunate or tragic outcomes. Genetics has been used as the basis for granting insurance coverage or employment or educational opportunity to some, while slamming the door on others. It has been used to set government policies such as immigration laws, providing a haven to some, while keeping others out. Recent history is riddled with deplorable and brutal events, the most extreme human abuses, that the perpetrators justified using "genetic" reasons.

The beliefs or excuses that were used as the basis of these policies were primitive, imperfect, or just plain wrong. Our knowledge of the genetic material, and of the ways genes act, has advanced since that time. With the new DNA tests, we can examine the DNA molecule and find out about individual genes using tools much more precise than ever before. Tests can detect a single gene that will bring on a severe (and expensive) illness. Tests can detect genes that provide information about the likelihood of later developing a chronic disease. There is little doubt that the new forms of DNA testing could be of interest to insurance companies, employers, schools, and government agencies. Questions arise:

Is anyone else entitled to have access to information about our genes? Can the DNA tests we take now be used later to discriminate against us? How much "genetic privacy" do we really have? Who will be permitted to gain access to our personal genetic information in the future?

A Grim Lesson from the Past: The "Eugenics" Movement

Discrimination directed against individuals and the labeling of whole groups of people as inferior has been a somber and enduring theme throughout all of human history. Since the time of the ancient Greeks, there was the idea that something tangible, "something in the blood," accounted for the similarities observed between parent and child and the differences between one family and the next. What this something was, and how it was passed along, was not known. By the end of the nineteenth century, support began to spread for the notion that, just as it was possible to select the best organisms for reproduction and improve the features of animals and plants, it could be possible to intervene to improve human heredity.

In 1883, this notion became codified in the term "eugenics" coined by Francis Galton, an illustrious British scientist and mathematician. Taken from the Greek for "well-born," eugenics was proposed by Galton as the means to improve the qualities of the human race. Those with good qualities should be encouraged to reproduce more abundantly. Those with inferior qualities should be discouraged from reproducing. Not surprisingly, the definition of "good qualities" always mirrored the attributes of the person or group making the distinction. Gaining entry to elite educational institutions, winning honors, and attaining high social status were all seen as having a purely hereditary basis. Curiously, social or economic factors that could account for these features were disregarded. (Perhaps not so curiously, since those promoting eugenic ideas were of course members of the privileged classes, their neglect of these other factors was self-serving.)

The recognition that heredity could be tied to physical units (soon to be called genes) came at the turn of the twentieth century, with the rediscovery of Mendel's laws. Supporters of eugenics could now point to a more concrete physical agent of heredity. It became possible to hold specific genes responsible for bringing about specific desirable or undesirable traits. Wherever they looked, eugenics enthusiasts saw a simple genetic basis for complex characteristics. Single genes provided for intelligence and for the love of going to sea. Single genes accounted for pauperism, feeblemindedness, prostitution, thievery, even insubordination. Nearly any social ill or frowned-upon behavior came to be ascribed to a gene. Looking back, it is easy to see how absurd these ideas were. The data on which they were based were spurious, supported by bigotry rather than biology. But it became convenient to believe that stubborn social problems could be blamed on the bearers of "bad genes" that were passed along by seemingly simple rules. In addition to some scientists, many politicians and other people in influential positions signed on as supporters of eugenic views.

The seeds of eugenics spread rapidly. They took hold in many countries in the soil of the prejudice, which is most fertile when times are hard. In the United States, eugenic ideas grew into efforts to restrict immigration from southern and central Europe in order to keep out people, especially Italians and Jews, considered genetically inferior. The Immigration Act of 1924 was written to favor the entry of immigrant groups from Great Britain and northwestern Europe; it restricted the admission of people coming from other parts of Europe, people regarded as genetically unsound. These restrictive quotas later had tragic consequences for people trying to escape Nazi savagery in the 1930s.

During a thirty-year period that started in 1907, eugenic ideas also drove the enactment of state laws that permitted the involuntary sterilization of people thought to have unfavorable genes. Ultimately, more than sixty thousand such sterilizations were carried out in over thirty states. Some of those sterilized were classified as "feebleminded." Some had behavior problems which brought them into state institutions. These included swearing, appearing unkempt, and (for women) being sexually active while unmarried. Most were just poor and uneducated and from broken families. The lack of education and the debilitating effects of poverty were ignored. The prevailing eugenic view was that all of these behaviors were caused by genes, and it was important to keep these genes from being passed on.

The worst excesses occurred in Nazi Germany. Here eugenic ideas, twisted together with a long festering hatred of minorities and fed by a political and economic crisis, fueled a chain of increasingly appalling events. Laws were enacted for the compulsory sterilization of people deemed unfit. More than four hundred thousand of these sterilizations were performed. This was followed by policies that permitted involuntary euthanasia, or "mercy killing," first of children with serious physical or mental illness, and then of adults. Some two hundred thousand people declared "unworthy of life" were put to death. And it ended in the abyss of genocide—the murder of six million Jews (including two million children) and millions of others (including homosexuals and Gypsies)—carried out in assembly lines of death at the concentration camps.

The eugenic policies of the first half of the twentieth century have long since been discredited. Many people who had first been supporters dissociated themselves early on as the inaccuracies, distortions, and downright stupidity of eugenic views became apparent. Many were turned off by the evils that resulted. The forced sterilizations, the "mercy" killings, and the enormity of the horrors of the Holocaust made the viciousness of these policies manifest and unacceptable. Although few of us can recite the details of the evils of the history of eugenics, there is a deep collective memory of that history that persists. To this day, the idea that our genes could somehow be held against us lurks in the shadows. This fear, along with the temptation in contemporary society to point to genes as the primary determinant of who we are and what we may become, makes us distinctly uneasy when decisions about genetic testing are being considered.

Genetic Testing and Insurance

Information about our genes could be of keen interest to others, particularly those who provide insurance. Companies that sell insurance—whether it is life, health, or disability insurance—base the rates for their plan on estimates of an applicant's current and future health status, as well as on estimates of the risks associated with the applicant's lifestyle activities (such as race-car driving or bungee jumping). The more likely it is that a person would die or be injured, the higher the price of the policy. To help them estimate these probabilities, insurance companies ask for your age, family history, and other relevant lifestyle information as part of the application process. They ask your physician for records outlining your current state of health and specifying any health problems you may be experiencing. Some companies require examinations conducted by their own physicians. Current problems are considered "pre-existing conditions" and may disqualify a person for insurance coverage or may result in a reduction of benefits for care related to that condition. At present, genetic information is used in a limited way, and questions usually concern disorders whose symptoms have already appeared or that may have affected your relatives.

The newest forms of genetic testing could provide companies with available additional information about whether, even though you are healthy now, you are susceptible to some major diseases that may shorten your life or that may be costly to treat. Insurers who got hold of such information would be able to incorporate that genetic prediction into their decision to approve a policy and in setting the premiums you would have to pay. It would also allow them to avoid what they call "adverse selection." Adverse selection occurs when someone who knows of an impending health problem buys large amounts of insurance in order to later collect handsomely from a policy toward which he or she would have paid in very little. This causes companies to lose money, which they make up by increasing the cost of premiums for other policy holders. This makes insurance coverage more expensive and, for some, unaffordable. In extreme cases, such financial losses might drive companies out of business.

Many consumer groups believe that insurance companies should not be allowed to demand genetic tests or gain access to the results of tests that have already been done. These consumers maintain that making genetic testing a condition for getting insurance would force many of them to acquire information that they have decided they do not want to have. Moreover, giving insurance companies access to previous genetic test results violates the privacy of other relatives; their genetic risks could become known to others without their knowledge or consent. Also, many object to the offensive practice of "cherry-picking," in which insurance companies try to limit coverage to only the very safest risks, thus maximizing their profits, and avoiding their industry's obligation to provide broad coverage. Genetic information might provide new opportunities for such industry abuse, and might deny essential coverage to many.

Genetic professionals are skeptical about the real value of genetic tests for an insurance company's calculations. They point out that there is far too little understanding of the long-term health effects any particular variation in the DNA may produce, or if the variation found means anything at all. Since genetic tests are imperfect predictors of a person's future health status, it would be inappropriate to consider the mere presence of a genetic variation as a pre-existing condition. Furthermore, they argue, penalizing people who are found to have a susceptibility gene makes no sense. It fails to take into account the beneficial changes people make in their lives in response to testing, changes that improve their health and lower their risk of developing illness. Motivated by their test results, people have quit smoking, increased exercising, modified their diet to include more fruits and vegetables, and begun to have regular medical checkups. Genetic professionals worry that consumers, fearful that a genetic test result could make them ineligible for insurance coverage, may be less likely to have the test and then to make these lifestyle changes. As a result, they will be less likely to be diagnosed early and less able to take advantage of treatments at the earliest stages of an illness when the treatments are most effective.

The appropriate handling of genetic information by insurance companies is not just a topic for debate. It is becoming a matter of real concern. Enough anecdotal reports have accumulated to show that genetic information has been used to deny some people health insurance completely, or to rule out specific types of coverage. Quite often, the reports reveal a significant lack of understanding by those in insurance organizations charged with making decisions. Many times the judgments made have been at odds with well-known genetic principles and with medical experience. People who are carriers of recessive genes, such as for sickle-cell anemia or cystic fibrosis, have been denied insurance by some companies, even though carriers are perfectly healthy and at no risk for those illnesses. The mere presence of a genetic variation has been ignorantly equated with illness by some insurers, even when there are no symptoms at all. Genetic disorders have been retroactively labeled a pre-existing condition and benefits have been denied. Naturally, there is apprehension that as scientists provide a larger repertoire of DNA tests which allow the recognition of more susceptibility genes, even more ill-founded decisions may be made.

In contrast to the growing evidence elsewhere of insurance company use (or misuse) of genetic information, the individuals who contributed to the present study reported relatively few problems with their health insurance coverage. Most have been covered by large group plans in which employees and family members are automatically covered. Some, facing high medical costs, have been able to use special insurance coverage provided with county, state, or federal assistance. Several people, anticipating problems they might face if they had to reapply for health insurance, said they felt locked in to their current job with its assured health plan. It was apparent to many of these consumers that, for the most part, insurance companies still have little or no knowledge of genetic disorders. One woman with Charcot-Marie-Tooth disease, a neurological disorder bearing the name of the three researchers who first identified the condition, had a claim rejected. She was told that her insurance plan did not provide any dental benefits! After she explained that "Tooth" was a person and not a body part, the claim was paid.

An insurance issue that was consistently noted by consumers is this: It took endless negotiation and discussion and hassle to sort payment matters out. The time it took to protest, explain, and provide extra documentation was extremely wearing for families caring for a child with a disability. One woman felt that dealing with the insurance company had become her "part-time job." For another couple, discussions with the insurance company sometimes took two hours a day. They were convinced that the insurance company was "stonewalling" them. Ultimately, the company paid up. But the time they lost, precious time away from their dying child, could not be restored. The adversarial tone that company representatives frequently adopt is particularly cruel and painful for parents who have already lost a child. In one case, the bills began to come in nearly three months after the death of a baby. "I didn't want to have to fight," explained the mother. "I thought it was something you should not have to worry about. I mean that is why you have insurance. I made the appropriate phone calls right after he died and was assured that it would all be taken care of. And yet here it all was. It was so disheartening." The bills were finally paid by the insurance plan, but at the cost of additional and unnecessary misery inflicted by the insurance settlement process.

The tensions between the insurance community on the one hand and the consumer and genetic professional communities on the other, about whether genetic information should be used, are proving difficult to resolve. Some state governments have stepped in and taken action to address aspects of the insurance issue. Private health insurance is seen as the form of insurance needing the most urgent attention. In the absence of a national health-care system that covers all citizens, the majority of consumers are dependent on meeting health-care costs through insurance plans provided by their employer or purchased on their own. The genetic testing provisions that have been developed vary widely from state to state. Some states restrict insurer access to genetic information for only a few disorders (such as for sickle-cell or Tay-Sachs). Other states, such as California and Wisconsin, have broader provisions which limit insurer access to genetic test results and prohibit *any* use of genetic tests during the application process. At the moment, no state regulation prevents insurers from using genetic information derived from sources *other* than tests—such as from family history or from comments on the medical record.

Consumers who want to find out the policies (if any) in force in their state will need to contact their state insurance commission. The location and phone number of the commission office can be found in the state government section in the telephone book, or through the National Association of Insurance Commissioners. The Alliance of Genetic Support Groups puts out a booklet, the *Health Insurance Resource Guide,* that contains useful information and advice for consumers seeking health insurance. Check the Appendix, Sections II and V, for ways to reach these organizations.

Several task forces have looked into these insurance questions. They have urged that genetic information *not* be used either for making decisions about health-coverage eligibility or in setting premiums. They point out that genetic information is superfluous, since insurance companies have developed sophisticated means of assessing risk using ordinary measures. The actuarial (statistical) data that the companies use to determine risk probabilities already incorporate risks of genetic illness.

There are a number of efforts under way at the federal level to establish a uniform policy for the use of genetic testing in insurance. This national policy would apply in all states and would replace the current patchwork of policies. It would also apply to self-funded insurance plans, plans set up by individual businesses to provide health care for their own employees. Self-funded plans now cover about half of the workforce in the United States. These plans are currently exempt from state regulation.

One initiative by the federal government is the Health Insurance Portability and Accountability Act (effective 1 July 1997). This act offers some protection to workers who change or lose their jobs. For a worker who is already covered in a self-funded employer plan or in a group health plan offered by a health insurer, it provides for the continuance of health insurance and it limits any waiting period imposed for a pre-existing condition. The act also restricts the use of genetic information in determining eligibility for insurance and in setting premium contributions. The effects of this bill, and the ways it can lead to protection for those who are not covered (self-employed, unemployed, or those not receiving benefits at work) remain to be seen.

Genetic Testing and the Workplace

Whether an office or a factory, or a bus or airplane or construction site, the workplace is another area of life into which genetic information can intrude. Genetic testing can become an issue in the workplace in two ways. It can be used by an employer with a self-funded health insurance plan to estimate what a job applicant's expected medical claims (or those of that person's family) might be. A company could then decide not to hire someone whom they think might have frequent claims or expensive treatments that could prove costly for the company's health plan. As described in the previous section, there are legal remedies being considered at the state and national levels that are intended to prevent genetic information from being used in this way.

Genetic testing could also be used to "predict" the future work performance of a job candidate. A genetic test showing that an applicant has a gene that predisposes to illness might be interpreted to mean the eventual reduction of that person's physical or mental ability to carry out a job (for instance, if heart problems or symptoms of Alzheimer's disease develop later). Or it might be interpreted to mean possible time lost from work at some point in the future. Genetic tests could be used to identify those who might be more susceptible to harmful reactions from certain chemicals found in the workplace environment. Any of these interpretations could be used as reasons to declare someone unsuitable for a job and to deny employment. For this kind of genetic discrimination, a remedy already exists in the form of a novel piece of legislation: the Americans with Disabilities Act.

Signed into law by President Bush on 26 July 1990, the Americans with Disabilities Act (the ADA) was the result of protracted efforts by people with disabilities to gain relief from the discrimination they faced in many areas of their lives. The law forbids discrimination in employment in any business or organization with more than fifteen employees, in public services (such as transportation, hotels, stores, restaurants), in state and local government services, and in telecommunications (for those who are deaf or blind). According to the law, a person is disabled if (1) he or she has an impairment—physical or mental—that substantially limits one or more of that person's major life activities; or (2) has a record of such impairment; or (3) is regarded as having such an impairment. In the workplace, employers are expected to focus on the ability of the applicant to do the job. Employers are expected to make "reasonable accommodation," if necessary, so that those with disabilities can carry out the basic job functions.

How does the ADA apply to genetic disorders and genetic tests? Individuals with an existing impairment which restricts their activities and which was brought on by a genetic disorder qualify as disabled according to the first criterion. They are covered by all the provisions of the ADA. Those who have been treated in the past for cancer or for a genetic disorder, and who are now symptom free, qualify under the second criterion. And in March 1995, the Equal Employment Opportunity Commission (EEOC, which enforces portions of the ADA) determined that the third criterion of "disabled" applies to those who suffer employment discrimination because of genetic information. Thus the ADA protects healthy persons who have had a genetic test that reveals a gene that will bring on a disorder at a later date or that predisposes them to a disorder. By itself, having such a gene does not render a person "disabled." It is only when information about bearing the gene has been used to discriminate against someone in the realm of employment (because the individual is now *regarded* as having an impairment) that the law can be invoked. This is the first strong governmental statement that it is unacceptable to use genetic information to deprive people of employment. However, the EEOC position is subject to review by the courts.

This means that potential employers cannot ask you about your medical history, past insurance claims, absenteeism caused by illness, or any types of medical treatments that you have used or are using. (Of course, interviewers sometimes verbally ask such illegal questions. There are prudent interview-taking techniques to deal with such questions without appearing confrontational.) Nor can medical examinations be requested in advance of making a job offer. Any required medical examinations can be carried out only *after* employment has been offered and only if such examinations are absolutely necessary and are mandatory for everyone who takes that job. An offer could be withdrawn only if the tests revealed that it would not be possible for a person to carry out the essential functions of the job. It is a violation of the ADA to withdraw a job offer based on genetic tests.

Even with its groundbreaking features, the ADA does not offer protection in every area. According to the law, the use of standard risk evaluation (underwriting) procedures by insurance companies does not constitute discrimination. So, though the costs of insurance cannot be a factor in the hiring process itself, insurers can refuse to cover a pre-existing condition and can exclude disabled employees from group health insurance.

Further, despite the ADA's strong stance against genetic testing as a condition of employment, it would seem that a niche for genetic tests could exist in the employment picture. There are some jobs for which strict standards—whether of strength, endurance, or reaction time—need to be met and to which the "reasonable accommodation" requirement of the ADA could not apply. Into this category might fall firefighters, police, airplane pilots, bus drivers, and others whose personal health directly affects their work in the public safety area. Employers may regard genetic tests as necessary to show whether or not an employee has hidden cardiovascular or muscle impairments. However, it is hard to see how genetic tests could be effective for this purpose. Except in very rare cases, the tests of strength, reaction time, heart function, and vision that are currently used at the time of hiring and periodically afterward would be far superior measures of a person's real ability to carry out a job than any vague hint that a genetic test result could provide.

There are jobs in many types of industrial environments in which workers may be exposed to high levels of chemicals. Genetic tests could be seen as a means of identifying workers who may be more susceptible to suffering harmful health effects from such chemical exposure. There are reports that some large industrial companies have, in fact, used genetic tests to detect defective forms of two or three genes associated with anemia or lung damage. It is not clear if such genetic studies are still being done. Evidence that workers with such genes are at higher risk is meager. It is possible that genetic tests may come along in the future that are better at predicting who may be most sensitive to chemical pollution in the workplace. Here too, all of those exposed, not only those found to be the most sensitive, will likely exhibit some kind of adverse effect. It would make sense and prove more cost-effective in the long run for companies to reduce chemical exposure and institute appropriate handling practices for all workers.

More information on the Americans with Disabilities Act can be obtained by contacting the Equal Employment Opportunities Commission, Office of Communications and Legislative Affairs, in Washington, D.C. The address and telephone numbers can be found in Section V of the Appendix.

Genetic Testing and Genetic Privacy

There are rising concerns that the new genetic tests might be the seed around which a resurgence of eugenic ideas and policies—a "new eugenics"—could crystallize. These are not idle worries. When testing for the sickle-cell anemia gene was first carried out in the early 1970s, it provided many lessons on the countless ways genetic test information can be misunderstood and misused. Those who are carriers of the sickle-cell gene are said to have "sickle-cell trait." But people with sickle-cell trait are not sick! Along with the recessive sickle-cell gene, individuals with sickle-cell trait carry a functional gene that ensures normal hemoglobin structure, sparing them hemoglobin-related health problems. (Carriers are also more resistant to malaria, should they be living in an environment where malaria occurs.) Nonetheless, the information about sickle-cell trait began to be insidiously placed into all kinds of official records.

As the word spread, it began to cause problems for people. In the U.S., most individuals with sickle-cell trait are African Americans. As in the heyday of eugenics, it was easy for bigotry to creep in. In some places, the test result harmed their ability to get insurance and to gain employment. Seeing the sickle-cell trait label in student files, some teachers misinterpreted this to mean that there was a learning impairment and they used genetics as a reason for excluding children from educational enrichment programs. The U.S. military prohibited men with sickle-cell trait from entering the Air Force Academy. Among other serious problems created by the sickle-cell gene testing programs were the indiscriminate spread of private genetic information and the damaging and totally unjustified denial of opportunity based on this information. In this new era of DNA testing, we would be foolish to ignore those grave mistakes from the recent past.

Many professional and consumer groups are calling for laws to protect the privacy of all genetic information. These calls are being heard at the state, national, and international levels. Though the proposals that have been advanced differ, they share some common features.

First it is generally held that genetic information, as any other medical information, should be confined to the physician/patient interaction. Confidentiality should not be breached unless the patient gives specific permission for the genetic information to be released. There is also general agreement that decisions about hiring, granting scholarships, and admission into school or job programs should be made on the basis of an applicant's own talent, skills, and record of accomplishment. Individuals should be judged solely on their credentials at the time of application. Concerns about possible future problems with vision, hearing, mobility, and other aspects of health, while potentially useful for the *individual* in forging his or her own life plans, should not be part of decisions made by third parties. Additionally, the conditions under which genetic information could be requested and used by others (such as the courts, employers, school officials, government agencies, and insurers) need to be limited and need to be carefully spelled out in any genetic-privacy policy or law.

Coming up with a set of rules for protecting genetic privacy will be difficult. Keeping genetic information private is a problem because keeping *any* medical information private is a problem. It has been estimated that more than fifty people (including secretaries, clerks, and pharmacists) may have ready access to a person's ordinary medical records. In a hospital setting, that figure climbs to nearly a hundred and fifty. The Medical Information Bureau in Massachusetts is a national storehouse of information, available to insurance companies, that has been gathered from previous applications for insurance. The increasing use of computers for record keeping raises concern about how genetic information is stored and how it could be found and used by others. Rules protecting privacy will need realistic procedures for carrying them out and will need to carry penalties that are effective in discouraging noncompliance.

Until such matters are resolved, many genetic professionals think it is prudent to warn their clients of the possibility that their personal genetic information could be used in ways they may not want. Deferring genetic testing until after insurance matters have been arranged may still not be enough to prevent misuse in other contexts later on. The Americans with Disabilities Act is a start, a shot across the bow of genetic injustice. Further action is needed to prevent individuals and groups from suffering genetic prejudice. It remains to be seen when such action will be taken. Consumers could help by urging their legislators to put this issue at the top of their agenda. Like Ebenezer Scrooge, we must be mindful of the ghost of eugenics past and banish the ghost of eugenics, in whatever shape it threatens to take, from our future.

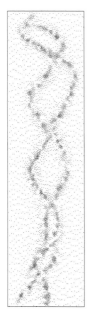

Chapter Seven

The Outlook for Future Genetic Tests and Treatments

There is no doubt that human gene research is proceeding at a vigorous pace. In laboratories around the world, scientists are actively exploring sections of the vast length of the railroad track of DNA that runs through every chromosome. They begin by studying families to find markers showing the general area along this track where the gene for a disorder is located. With the aid of many types of searching techniques, they proceed to narrow down the region until, finally, they find where the individual gene resides. The DNA message for the gene from unaffected and affected family members is then deciphered to identify places within the gene where disruptions or changes have occurred that cause the disorder. There is the expectation that such detailed knowledge will tell us not only what the gene normally does, but also how to develop better tests, improve treatments, and ultimately even cure the genetic disorder.

For many consumers, a report of new progress in genetic research may be far more than a newsworthy item of momentary interest. Studies under way on the scientific front can both ease and complicate their crucial life decisions. People concerned about an inherited disorder for which the gene is still not known, or for which treatments do not yet exist, often find themselves caught between what medical science can offer them right now and what may be just around the corner. Should they put off having children until genetic tests come along that could identify those with the flawed gene in their family? How long do they dare delay? Or should they go ahead and have children, hoping that researchers will be able to come up with effective new treatments that will be ready just when they are needed? How reasonable is it to hope for these things?

In the following pages, we will look at what the record has been in finding genes and what effect the now-underway massive "Human Genome Project" may have on this process. We will examine how long it can take from the time the search begins until the gene is finally flushed out, and we will see how long it can take from the time a gene is identified until reliable tests or therapies emerge. We will also see how consumers have become active partners in the scientific enterprise, helping to improve the chances that progress will be made in areas of most direct concern to them.

The Direction and Speed of Research to Find Genes

KEY INDICATORS

Of the estimated one hundred thousand different genes on all the human chromosomes, over five thousand are associated with the relatively rare single-gene disorders, and a growing number are now recognized as having some role in the relatively more common health disorders. This means that not every gene for every disorder can command the full attention of the scientific community. A major element influencing the choice of which genes get selected for study is a practical one: the availability of funds to permit that research to proceed. Funding enables scientists to pursue research. Conversely, lack of funding inhibits it.

Obtaining money for research is very difficult. Researchers often spend a large part of their time pursuing adequate financial support for their work. The federal government, through the National Institutes of Health (NIH), is the largest supplier of grants for the conduct of medical research. Unfortunately, federal funding for research on inherited disorders is greatly limited by the competing demands on the NIH budget. The NIH is responsible for many health matters, such as providing better forms of child health care, dealing with problems of substance abuse, extending the understanding of nutrition, and improving treatments for debilitating diseases.

Because federal funding is in short supply, research dollars must also be sought from other private-sector sources such as the pharmaceutical industry and the biotechnology industry. In the private sector, the emphasis tends to be on support for studies of the common disorders, since these would yield a potentially large and lucrative market for any tests or treatments that emerge from the research. As a result, research on disorders that affect relatively few individuals may suffer from insufficient financial support and may be overlooked entirely.

Even if financial support is obtained, success in tracking down genes is not assured. A number of factors intervene. Particularly important is the *degree of cooperation* that can be developed among the various investigators. Competition is as much a fact of life in science as it is elsewhere in society. It has often been asserted that scientific work can proceed most rapidly when different rival groups compete against each other as they race toward the same goal. That way, it is felt, each group will intensify its separate efforts, lured on by the desire for acclaim and the professional rewards that often go along with being the first to report a successful outcome.

However, for this type of research a different mode, one emphasizing collaboration among investigators, actually produces results more quickly. There are many recent examples of this. In the search for the Huntington disease, cystic fibrosis, ataxia telangiectasia, and breast cancer genes, investigators chose to put competitiveness aside and form consortiums to exchange information freely about DNA markers, probes, dead ends, and the like. This prevented a wasteful duplication of effort. Each participant could pick a promising piece of chromosomal turf and inspect it thoroughly, knowing that no matter where the gene was finally found, all would share in the success.

This mode of interaction is beginning to take hold in the genetic research community. Collaborative arrangements are now being formed among groups investigating the genetic basis of many different human disorders.

Researchers are quick to point out that formal collaborations have their problems too. Collaborations sometimes hamper the progress of those laboratories that, for political or other reasons, are excluded. The greater difficulty in getting credit for one's own ideas when part of a large team may be a disincentive to some researchers. And collaborations occasionally have a tendency to break apart just as the members are closing in on their quarry.

One technique used by geneticists to help pinpoint the target gene is to refer to the gene "map." Such a map shows the location of human genes along each chromosome much in the same way that a train map shows the location of towns along each rail line. Researchers take the gene map (as it is known at the present time) and scan the section where linkage studies have placed the gene. They do this to see what genes are already known to be located in that section of the chromosome. One of these genes could be the site of the genetic flaw. The presence of such "candidate" genes in that section of the chromosome improves the odds of a successful search, since the target gene is *either* a candidate gene *or* an as-yet-unknown gene. If that section of the gene map contains several known genes, then the search may succeed quickly. However, if it contains few or no known genes, then there may be no likely suspects to study. The target gene, in such a case, is a still-unidentified gene in the chromosome section of interest. In this situation, laborious and tedious (and time-consuming) techniques for examining the DNA must be used. Thus the more genes there are that have been identified and located on the human gene map, the better are the chances that any search will succeed.

The search for the gene that causes one form of Marfan syndrome, a disorder of connective tissue, was helped by the candidate gene approach. Linkage studies had narrowed down the location of the Marfan syndrome gene to a section of chromosome 15. On the map of that section was a gene that produced a protein called fibrillin.

Fibrillin is a component of the structural support system of many parts of the human body. The possibility that fibrillin was related to some forms of Marfan syndrome now demanded attention. When it was found that individuals with Marfan syndrome also had mutations in the fibrillin gene, it was possible to conclude that these mutations were responsible for the disorder, establishing that gene's connection to Marfan syndrome.

Overall then, these are encouraging signs: a good level of financial support, the willingness of research teams to cooperate rather than compete, and the gene's location in a well-mapped section of the chromosome. However, in estimating how long it may take to find a gene, we need to keep in mind that any gene search can be hindered or derailed by other factors. For instance, the region of the chromosome where the gene resides may possess some structural barriers, based on the pattern of DNA bases, that are hard to cross. Peculiar chromosomal geography on the tip of chromosome 4 created many problems for the researchers who were trying to nail down the Huntington disease gene. The search for a gene for adult polycystic kidney disease was slowed by the presence of several similar (though nonfunctional) genes in the same region as the true target gene. For a long time these acted as decoys, jamming and deflecting the researchers' genetic radar. Searches will be more complicated, and slower, if genes are positioned in difficult chromosomal terrain.

Other factors can block progress in finding the target gene. Linkage studies (which approximately locate the gene) are hard or impossible to do when the disorder is so rare that there are too few families to study. Linkage studies can also be confused when a malfunction in any one of several different genes can lead to the same disorder, so that the various forms cannot be distinguished from one another. Also, if there is a significant environmental component that influences the way the gene functions, it will take more time and effort to identify the gene.

How long does it take, this research journey to locate a gene? For the Huntington disease gene, it took ten years from the time that the first closely linked DNA marker was found in 1983 to the time that the gene itself and the mutation within it were found. It took nine years to find the gene for adult polycystic kidney disease, once its placement on the tip of chromosome 16 was recognized. It took seven years to find the gene on chromosome 10 for one type of multiple endocrine neoplasia (MEN2A). The approximate location of BRCA1, the breast cancer susceptibility gene, was found in 1990. The gene itself was found four years later. Another breast cancer susceptibility gene, BRCA2, was found in 1995. It took one year.

It certainly looks as if the time lag (the time between the first sniffing out of a gene's presence and the actual identification of the gene) is shrinking. It took a decade to find the Huntington disease gene because it was one of the first disorders studied with the new DNA searching procedures. The "infrastructure"—the necessary techniques, equipment, and means of analysis—was not yet in place. It had to be created as the search went along. Over the years, a vast arsenal of tools to track down and identify genes has been developed. What was incredibly difficult to do just a few years ago is now becoming much easier. Recent searches are the beneficiaries of the earlier ones. Still, given all the confounding factors we have described above, it is hard to estimate how long any particular search will take. Researchers suggest that, with current technologies, consumers should expect it to take at least five years to find a gene.

Identifying the target gene does not bring with it the certainty that a genetic test will quickly be possible. After the gene is found, there will be a further lag while investigators work to understand which variations in the gene are important and which aren't. The longer the gene, the more DNA there is to investigate. For some target genes, there may be a few common mutations that cause the disorder in many (sometimes most) families. When this happens, direct genetic tests can be designed to see if an individual possesses one of those mutations. If, on the other hand, many different mutations occur and each family has its own unique form, then a linkage test will probably be the main form of genetic testing. Linkage tests are also the only form of testing that can be used while gene searchers are still closing in on the target gene. Making sure that tests are accurate, reproducible from laboratory to laboratory, and produce few false positive or false negative results adds to the time (from months to a year or more) before a test becomes available.

THE HUMAN GENOME PROJECT

A major research project has been accelerating the search for genes by providing researchers with an enormous store of information about chromosome geography. Rather than limiting searches to the region around a few target genes, scientists have organized in a large collaborative effort to seek out every human gene. The word "genome" describes the *total* genetic material contained in a full set of chromosomes of an organism. The work being carried out to locate, map, and decipher the chemical structure of all human genes is known as the Human Genome Project.

We saw earlier that the more we know about the human gene map, the easier it is to find a target gene. Thus the completion of the gene map should prove to be of great benefit to genetic testing. The complete gene map will come out as one key product of the Genome Project. The other key product, full knowledge of the human genome, will include still more information, since it will even spell out the details of the DNA base-pair structure within each gene.

This enormously ambitious project began in the mid-1980s, when a few researchers suggested that instead of laboriously filling in the gene map one gene at a time, a massive effort could be undertaken to find the positions of all the human genes on each of the 23 chromosome pairs. Going even further, they envisioned that it would be possible to determine the precise order or sequence of *all* three billion DNA base pairs contained within the human genome! Original estimates were that it would take fifteen years, at a cost of about three billion dollars, to mobilize the scientific teams that could reach this fantastic objective. Before long, this bold—and controversial—proposal took hold in the scientific community. In 1989, the U.S. Congress authorized funds to begin this project under the joint auspices of the National Institutes of Health and the Department of Energy. Other countries, including France, the U.K., and Japan, have initiated their own similar projects in what has now become a worldwide enterprise.

The research teams working on the Human Genome Project are exceeding their original timetable. Maps of each chromosome containing numerous DNA markers, landmarks along the chromosomes, have been produced. Tiny chunks of DNA representing pieces of all of the chromosomes, each possessing its own specific landmarks, are stored away in various forms. Collectively, these chromosome pieces constitute a library of human DNA. Researchers are moving full-steam ahead to work out the precise sequence of the four bases in the DNA in each of these pieces. By early in the twenty-first century, the entire structural record of human DNA should be known. It should then be relatively easy to know where all the genes are. This structural record should also be a valuable tool for working out the precise function of genes and for figuring out how they may go awry.

Even before all this work is completed, the task of finding specific target genes should be greatly simplified. Researchers will be spared having to search everywhere along a seemingly endless, and sometimes desolate, DNA track. As soon as family studies reveal a DNA marker linked to a target gene, researchers can use that marker as a reference point and extract the chromosome section containing the marker from the chromosome library. They can then concentrate their search for the target gene on that small section of the chromosome. The time spent identifying a target gene associated with hereditary illness should be reduced from years to, perhaps, just months.

The Speed and Direction of Research into Treatments

Optimism in the research community about prospects for locating genes and developing tests to find their flaws is not matched by optimism that treatments for genetic disorders will be found as quickly.

Up until now, success in developing treatments has been uneven. Traditionally, for single-gene disorders, the emphasis has been on trying to fix the problems that occur after the gene malfunctions. The approaches that have come out of the laboratory and into the medical setting have involved restricting certain foods in the diet, using drugs to correct chemical imbalances, supplying missing substances, replacing damaged organs with healthy ones, and correcting by means of surgical procedures. The degree of effectiveness of these treatments varies from person to person and from illness to illness. Some current treatments offer only partial relief of symptoms. Many carry with them unpleasant side effects or exorbitant costs. Most require a life-long commitment.

For the more prevalent multifactorial disorders, treatments have also concentrated on controlling symptoms with drugs and surgery. These have worked well for some conditions and poorly, or only tem-porarily, for others. The medical profession has less experience in trying to counter the effects of a damaged gene in these cases, since it is only recently that the genetic component of these disorders has even been appreciated.

Finding out what a gene does (or fails to do when it malfunctions) is no guarantee that a treatment will soon follow. The fact that the oxygen-carrying protein of the red blood cells is altered in sickle-cell anemia has been known for over forty years. Only now, after decades of research, are promising treatments in sight for sickle-cell anemia. This is not an isolated example. Even when the protein that a gene makes has been identified and can be produced in quantity in the laboratory, it has not been possible to use that protein to correct a hereditary dis-order. How to get the normal protein into the tiny recesses of the cells (in the part of the body where it needs to function) is a problem that has stubbornly resisted solution.

The focus of scientific interest is now shifting from the gene prod-uct to the gene itself. The most widely publicized treatment of this type is called "gene therapy."

Gene therapy has long been dreamt of as the ultimate magic bullet for defeating genetic disease. The idea of gene therapy is to correct genetic illness at its very root by placing the normal gene into the DNA of people who have inherited a flawed version. Restoring the normal genetic makeup would provide people with the capacity to produce the normal protein. Function would be restored, and people would be freed from the need to be continually treated for the problems inflicted by the flawed gene. What is turning gene therapy from fantasy into reality is a group of new techniques that allow a specific gene to be extracted out of the bulk of DNA and to be mass produced or "cloned" in the laboratory. Many of these techniques are the very same ones that have been perfected by researchers engaged in gene mapping. By the end of 1996, nearly two hundred experiments trying out various types of human gene therapy were under way in the United States, with numerous others taking place around the world. Most of these experiments were not aimed at addressing inherited disease but at developing new ways of treating cancer and AIDS. However, several have been directed at genetic disorders such as cystic fibrosis, Gaucher disease, Severe Combined Immunodeficiency (SCID-ADA disease), and a few others.

There has been a lot of hype surrounding these first attempts at gene therapy. As a result, many individuals have been misled into thinking that gene therapy is available for all genetic illnesses. One woman, who carries the gene for hemophilia, went ahead and became pregnant, fully anticipating that when her son was born he could be treated with the gene therapy she had heard so much about in the press. Other parents, reading about preliminary attempts to perform gene therapy for cystic fibrosis, had also come to believe that a proven therapy exists. All these parents were astonished to learn that there is still no gene therapy for hemophilia or for cystic fibrosis.

Consumers need to be aware that, as exciting and promising as gene therapy is, it is still in its very earliest stages. Daunting difficulties confront the researchers. It is not enough just to be able to produce many copies of a gene in a test tube. The gene must be introduced into the right cells. A gene for muscle function needs to be inserted into a muscle cell, and not into the liver, brain, or anywhere else. Once inside a cell, the gene must function properly. It must direct the production of its protein in the correct amount and at the appropriate time, and not work in an unbridled, erratic fashion. Researchers are still struggling to make gene therapy work. Until the problems are solved, gene therapy is not an option. There are no estimates for how long it might take to make it one. For any particular inherited illness, it could be years off.

There is another line of research, studies using animals as models for human disease, that could yield its own bonanza of new treatments. Animal models can be used to work out various experimental treatments and look for those which show the most potential before those same treatments are tried on humans. Some animals have genes that correspond, in some cases quite closely, to human genes. Mutations in those genes can give rise to illnesses in the animals that resemble those of humans. The diabetic mouse is one such example. Another type of model results from the ability of investigators to use genetic and reproductive technologies to construct animals that have a particular genetic makeup. "Knockout" mice, missing a single gene, and "transgenic" organisms, which are given an additional human gene, are produced in this way. There is, for instance, a transgenic mouse that expresses one of the mutant human genes for the early-onset form of Alzheimer's disease. This mouse exhibits structural brain changes that are similar to those in people with Alzheimer's. Studies using this type of mouse could provide an efficient way to distinguish effective drugs (drugs that prevent these structural changes and preserve brain function) from useless drugs.

Researchers are trying to refine and improve existing treatments and are eagerly searching for new ways to treat genetic illness. They are confident that some of these lines of work will pan out in the long term. In the short term, the prospects for finding effective treatments are *not* as good as the prospects for finding the responsible genes. While finding the gene can help direct research toward treatments and cures, it is only a first step toward that goal. Consumers need to temper their faith in the inevitability of medical progress with the awareness that treatments or cures may *not* come along in time to be of use to them. Hoping for a cure is fine, but counting on one is unwise.

Consumers as Partners in the Research Process

To the casual observer, the world of science appears impenetrable. It has its own highly technical language, unique habits of work, spaces filled with strange devices, and even its own form of dress—the lab coat.

Science seems to be cutting a giant swath through modern history—moving like a juggernaut, impervious to any outside influence. On closer inspection, however, it becomes apparent that this view is wrong. In reality, the world of science is very firmly rooted to the society in which it operates. After all, the questions that captivate scientific interest tend to be tied in with what is happening in the world at large. Scientists are stimulated in their thinking by the concerns and needs they see around them. The funds to fuel their work come from *outside* the scientific community, from governments, businesses, foundations, and other groups that typically want to have a certain set of problems pursued. Researchers must convince such patrons that their projects are worthy of support and must tailor projects to match the agendas of their potential donors.

These bonds between science and society are especially strong in the field of medical genetics. Here, to carry out its work, the research community is dependent on consumers and their families. The study of human genes simply would not be possible without the participation of those family groups in which there are genetic variations that can bring about illness. It is only through the study of such groups that scientists can begin to unravel details about gene function. Furthermore, laboratory investigations require an irreplaceable human resource: blood samples donated by affected and unaffected family members from which DNA can be extracted. With the blood samples, it becomes possible to determine a linkage pattern and find DNA markers that confine the search to a very small section of a chromosome. These same samples then enable researchers to close in on and identify the target gene. With the blood samples, a nameless gene on the gene map of the Human Genome Project can be connected to a real disorder. And, of course, new genetic tests and proposed treatments need, for their validation, the cooperation of research subjects from families with affected members. A partnership between the research and consumer communities is essential if progress is to be made in genetic medicine.

Usually the initiative for research comes from the scientists. However, there are several ways in which consumers can become more active

partners in this relationship. In doing so, consumers gain the opportunity to energize the research process and to influence what new areas
researchers will explore.

JOINING OR FORMING VOLUNTARY HEALTH ORGANIZATIONS

One extremely fruitful course of action has come from people who were
disappointed by an insufficient number of research programs on their
family's genetic disorder. Banding together, they have established
organizations to raise awareness among researchers and to generate
funds—two key ingredients for scientific work.

This type of consumer involvement has been effective in triggering interest and channeling research into new areas. One striking
example of this kind of lay-led activism were the efforts undertaken
by relatives of individuals stricken with Huntington disease. Groups
formed by the families of Woody Guthrie and Leonore Sabin Wexler
provided impetus to the study of Huntington disease, when little or
none had previously existed. This effort has had extraordinary success. The gene for Huntington disease was located and tests for the
mutation were developed. Not only have crucial advances relating to
Huntington disease resulted, but new concepts and techniques have
been created that benefit other areas of human genetic research.

In a similar fashion and for identical reasons, many other organizations have been formed when people whose lives had been touched
by a genetic disorder have banded together. Abbey Meyers, president
of the National Organization for Rare Disorders (NORD), notes, "There
are hundreds and hundreds of groups, and all of them really started
around a kitchen table." With the strength that comes in numbers, they
have found ways to raise money, to attract the interest of researchers,
to lobby for greater government support, and to funnel some of the funds
they have raised into projects of their own choosing. In a growing number of cases, members of these organizations have secured places on
government advisory panels that help allocate research funds.

In Section II of the Appendix is a list of umbrella agencies that consumers can contact to see if a voluntary health organization already
exists that matches their interests. If one does, they may want to

assist in its efforts. If none matches their interests, these same agencies can still provide information on how to get a new group started. One parent has summed up the reasons for her activism, "You can't just sit back and hope for a discovery. You have to make it happen." And they do.

ENROLLING IN REGISTRIES

Researchers endeavoring to study genetic disorders face a very practical problem. In order to be able to carry out their work, they need to have access to individuals and families who have these disorders. How can they do this when many disorders are relatively rare and when families are scattered all over the country?

One way that has been effective is to establish a *registry* of families with a particular medical condition or genetic disorder. The registry collects information on many different families. It keeps track of affected members, as well as those who are at risk. It provides a valuable database, giving researchers a sense of the different patterns of a disease's progression and feedback about the current treatments that seem to produce the most benefit. A registry can also further new research by matching up researchers with the population of subjects most appropriate for their investigations. Families in which there are several affected individuals are especially important for genetic studies.

Registries have been set up by medical researchers, by clinical research centers, and by lay organizations. The International Long QT Syndrome Registry, now officially based at the University of Rochester, had its beginnings in an informal registry started in the late 1970s by physicians wishing to learn more about certain heart rhythm anomalies. The Hereditary Hearing Impairment Registry was established in 1993 at the Boys Town National Research Hospital in Omaha. The Foundation Fighting Blindness in Baltimore has had a registry since 1989. Registries can be organized around single-gene disorders (such as the Metabolic Information Network in Dallas), multifactorial disorders (the National High Risk Registry for Breast Cancer at the Strang Cancer Prevention Center in New York City), and disorders whose genetic component is unclear (the National Registry for Familial Primary Pulmonary Hypertension at Vanderbilt University Medical Center). Wherever located and however organized, their major purpose is to help further research efforts.

These and other registries have already proven their worth in advancing research into the causes and treatments of genetic disorders. Consumers who want to become part of a registry will generally be sent a questionnaire asking them for personal and family information. In some cases they will be asked to provide medical records, or to authorize the registry to obtain information from their doctors. Because concerns about confidentiality always haunt any collection of personal medical information, consumers should first verify how the material they supply will be handled and how it will be updated. They should ask who will have access to their records. Those responsible for the registry should explain the procedures they will follow before they release information to researchers. They need to spell out how they will prevent unauthorized use by insurance companies or others. Some registries have obtained a "certificate of confidentiality," issued by the U.S. Department of Health and Human Services. Such a certificate protects researchers from ever being compelled to release information about a registry participant to anyone else, including courts, insurance companies, and employers.

STORING DNA SAMPLES

Blood and tissue from which to extract DNA are key resources in gene research. The storing of blood samples, in anticipation of their later use for some research purpose, can be of critical importance to future investigators. The inability to obtain such samples can make it impossible for some research to proceed. This problem often confounds the study of late-onset disorders because older affected members have already died. With a stored sample, the link is kept to an individual who may no longer be alive but whose DNA may be a reservoir of vital genetic clues.

For the most part, the storage of blood samples of individuals with disorders has been carried out by physicians and investigators in research laboratories, so that samples of DNA are available whenever they are ready to make use of them. The laboratory stores these samples as part of its research inventory. (The French Human Genome Project in Paris is collecting blood samples in Europe from families with rare genetic defects.) There are now commercial laboratories that collect and store blood samples for a fee that consumers themselves pay. Consumers arrange with these laboratories to keep samples, in case they are ever needed in the future for genetic testing of relatives. The samples may also be made available for later use in research, if permission is given.

It is important to keep in mind that it may be years before such samples are needed. The storage of samples does not mean that they will be examined immediately. Investigators cannot predict which problems they will be working on and which areas of study will be the most productive. Consumers should discuss with the research laboratory just how it anticipates making use of their samples. The forms which accompany the donation of the sample should describe how consumer privacy will be protected. The forms should also state whether the investigators plan to share with the sample donors any new information they acquire when the sample is used. For instance, if a mutation is found in their DNA, will they be told? Most families will want to check to see whether their stored DNA could be made available to other relatives. Andrew and Donna Stone, whose story has been told in Chapters One and Four, could not have had prenatal testing for spinal muscular atrophy if they had not taken the precaution of storing away a blood sample from Melissa, their first child, before she died. It was only through the linked markers found in Melissa's DNA that the prenatal linkage test at their next pregnancy could be interpreted.

PARTICIPATING IN RESEARCH STUDIES

The most visible way to contribute to the growth of knowledge is to become a research subject in scientific investigations. Consumers can learn of these studies from their physicians, from voluntary health organization newsletters, from a genetic registry, and from articles in the press. The nature of the participation will vary with the goals of each project. In some, the only involvement may be the contribution of a blood sample. In others, the subjects may be tested more extensively and may be examined periodically over months or years. Where experimental treatments are being tried, the procedures may be more invasive.

There is no question that research studies are the lifeline of science and medicine. But no one should consent to become a research subject without carefully considering the whole spectrum of risks and benefits of each particular project. What a person finds an acceptable balance of benefits and risks in one study may not hold for another study.

There is a period preceding any research study during which the investigators—or members of their staff—should be meeting with each prospective subject. They should describe, in nontechnical terms, what they are trying to learn and what will be expected of each person who takes part. Prospective subjects need to find out what the risks are as well as the benefits. Risks may vary from brief physical discomfort to more severe complications; from minor financial costs of travel to the laboratory, to having to pay medical expenses should there be a research-related injury. Benefits can range from the accumulation of general knowledge that will help others in the future, to the possibility of a specific improvement in genetic testing or treatment that can be of direct and immediate help to the research subject.

To avoid false hopes or expectations, subjects need to find out just what information, if any, they can expect to get back from the investigators. Will subjects be given any word about what was discovered? Will subjects be informed of any genetic information about them that is acquired in the course of the study? Which member of the study team should be contacted if the subject has questions later on? These aspects should be addressed *before* anyone signs a form giving his or her consent to participate. A pamphlet of advice to potential subjects of research, *Informed Consent: Participation in Genetic Research Studies,* can be obtained from the Alliance of Genetic Support Groups. (Its address is in Section II of the Appendix.)

The road to research success is not a straight one, nor are the steps along the way obvious. Not every important question is ripe for the answering. Sometimes the answering must await the development of new techniques or methods of analysis. Sometimes an advance in one area is spurred on by new understanding coming from work in a completely different area. The "war on cancer" of the 1970s poured large sums of money and resources into cancer research, yet yielded little. But studies on other illnesses, including the rare genetic disease ataxia telangiectasia, have provided substantial—and unexpected—insights into how a gene can contribute to cancer. As we have seen, the time it takes to identify a target gene and devise tests to track down troublesome changes in it is highly variable. Successful therapies are even more elusive. Researchers and consumers need to persevere in their partnership for a long period of time.

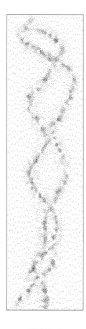

Chapter Eight

Nurturing the Genetic Grapevine

"There is nobody lonelier than the parent of a child just diagnosed with a genetic disorder."

"This is a very devastating thing and you are out there alone."

"There is no mechanism to 'welcome' parents into the situation. Getting a diagnosis like this turns you into a different social citizen and there is not any support."

"You have to be willing to go and do a little digging for information. There is no one out there to do it for you."

These are comments by people who have just learned that they or their child has a genetic disorder. At first glance, the heartfelt cry of unassisted aloneness may be surprising. After all, the diagnosis of a genetic disorder, or the news that one may be possible in the future, is almost always made somewhere within the walls of the medical community. It would seem that the vast resources of that community could easily be marshaled to provide information and help to those who need it.

In matters of illness, present-day society subscribes to what may be called the "medical model." The physician is the source of expert knowledge about disorders and their treatments. The relationship between physician and client (or patient), established in the office or examining room, allows each to be known to the other and each to interact directly with the other. Questions can be addressed. Mistaken ideas corrected. Choices evaluated. Decisions made. The physician acts as the point person, coordinating and overseeing a response to the diagnosis. It is the physician who arranges for whatever further tests are needed and who initiates any necessary contact with medical specialists, physical therapists, psychologists, dietitians, or others whose knowledge and skills could be useful. All efforts are directed toward achieving the best possible outcome for each individual patient.

If this medical model functions as it's supposed to and things work this way, then why is it that people facing a genetic illness feel so isolated? Why do they feel as if they have been cast adrift and left to fend for themselves to find the information and the assistance they need? One reason (as we have noted in Chapter Three) is that most physicians are simply *not* experts when it comes to genetic matters. Many are not informed on the subject. Genetics gets neglected. All too often, consumers are not referred to the experts, the genetic professionals who provide explanations and who know if genetic tests are available.

Another reason that the medical model is inadequate for genetic illness is that more than just one individual is involved. Genes run in families. With a genetic illness, it may be that relatives of the affected person have inherited the same genes. They or their children could be at risk for similar health problems. Except in rare circumstances, it is left to the person who receives the diagnosis, or who has the genetic counseling, to share what he or she has learned with other family members and to let them know about their possible risk. This responsibility applies, as well, when linkage testing is being done. There the relative seeking the genetic information is the one who must line up the other family members when their blood samples are needed. Thus it is a family member, not the physician (or even the genetic professional), who becomes the point person in the spread of genetic information. One woman who was in the process of alerting her siblings to a possible genetic problem was quite worried. "I don't know much," she remarked, "believe me." Unless others in her family opt to follow up on their own with a doctor or genetic counselor, almost all their information will come from her, and sometimes at second or third hand.

Thus, there is an important pathway for transmitting genetic information, one that is outside of the medical community. I call this the genetic grapevine. This pathway winds through families, from one member to the next, alerting people to the possibility of risk and indicating the methods available to determine that risk. This grapevine may function over many years. Family members, too young to be included at first, grow up and start to think about having their own children. Others, unconcerned at first, grow older and may begin to worry about possible changes in their own health. As their interest rises, relatives often turn to the family genetic grapevine as their primary source of information.

The genetic grapevine is not only a reality, it is a necessity. Consumers searching for genetic information cannot rely exclusively on medical sources. Medical sources can be ill-informed. Genetic professionals may be hard to find or not affordable. The medical community has no mechanism in place to locate past patients to tell them that research efforts have identified new genes and produced new tests. And, frankly, all the expertise does *not* reside in the medical community. Rich veins of information and insight on genetic matters exist elsewhere, particularly in families who have firsthand knowledge of genetic illness.

There are a number of resources that consumers can use to enrich their genetic understanding and keep up with new findings in research and treatment. Having information that is accurate and up-to-date is important not only for the individuals who seek it out for themselves; it is also important for the others in their family network who will learn of it through them. As we see below (and in the Appendix), the genetic grapevine can be nourished and reinforced with information in many different ways.

Public and Medical Libraries

Many consumers have sought information on their own by going to the traditional places where reference materials are collected. In their local libraries and, for some, in medical libraries, they have located books and articles that pertain to the genetic disorder of interest to them. In addition to their own holdings, libraries have computer links to other libraries and to databases of reference sources. MEDLINE®, an index of current medical periodicals, is one such database that can help locate relevant items in the medical literature. Reference librarians can be enlisted to help the consumer use these computer databases to look for needed information. Once books or articles in medical journals are identified, arrangements can be made to borrow the books from distant libraries or obtain photocopies of the articles.

There are difficulties in using the medical literature as the starting point for a search for information. Materials aimed at scientists and physicians may be so technical that they will be very hard to understand. The conclusions presented may have been supplanted by more recent studies or by more representative studies done on a broader sample. The text can be cold and, by emphasizing the most extreme aspects of an illness, brutal to read. One father discovered that the medical encyclopedia he had turned to for information on his son's Duchenne muscular dystrophy "was not a nice place to find out" about the disorder. Unless there is someone who can assist in interpreting the terms and ideas, it can be extremely perplexing for consumers to read these materials on their own.

Articles that have appeared in the popular press may be helpful, and reference guides (for example, the *Reader's Guide to Periodic Literature*) can be used to find such articles. Because these types of articles are written for a general audience, they will be the most understandable. They may, however, be brief, out of date, or overstate the significance of new research findings. Still, such articles can be informative and a good place to start. Consumers have found helpful reports in the science section of the *New York Times,* in the medical section of the *Washington Post,* and in the health column of the *Wall Street Journal.*

Lay-Led Health Organizations

The groups formed by individuals and family members most directly concerned with a particular genetic disorder are a valuable source of information for consumers. These groups, also known as voluntary (or volunteer) health organizations, carry out a variety of activities. Many of these activities are centered on providing educational materials (including such items as pamphlets and videotapes) that explain the nature of the disorder. These materials often serve as a good general introduction. Most of these groups also send out, on a regular basis, newsletters with articles that supplement the basic materials with the most recent research findings. These updates are useful indicators of the range of current tests and treatments. Often these groups are in close touch with researchers and clinicians, who serve as board members and consultants for them. Thus they are in a position to provide interpretations of new findings and to comment knowledgeably on the usefulness of possible new treatments. Some groups, as discussed in Chapter Seven, raise money to promote more research on their genetic condition.

Depending on their size and budget, these organizations may be able to assist consumers in other ways. They may direct affected individuals and their families to specialists and to an array of health-care services. One very large organization, the Muscular Dystrophy Association, provides services through its own clinics established at medical centers around the country. Most lay organizations assist in organizing peer support groups. Some organizations maintain registries (as described in Chapter Seven) to assist in research efforts, and several have worked with genetic counseling units to develop procedures for the way genetic testing will be handled. They act as advocates on behalf of people with genetic disorders, when insurance, education, and relevant government policies are being debated. Many of these organizations plan educational meetings which provide their members a review of the latest research.

There are many voluntary health organizations. They have headquarters throughout the country. As these organizations grow, they open branches in different regions. Sometimes smaller groups spin off to focus on one particular form of the genetic disorder. An efficient way to find the appropriate group is to begin by contacting one of the national coalitions. A list of such coalitions can be found in Section II of the Appendix.

The Internet

Recent developments in computers and in technologies that link computers with one another across long distances have opened up access to a treasure trove of information. Materials stored on computers in one location can easily be made available to people at other locations via a vast set of networks known as the Internet. The name "information superhighway" is used to describe this new system of communication and information transfer. At first, the travelers on the information superhighway were almost exclusively scientists. But now, consumers everywhere own their own computers and, with the use of a modem, they, too, are able to link their home computer to the Internet. (People who do not have the necessary equipment can use the computers and Internet-searching systems provided for patrons at many public libraries.) As a result, consumers can have access to many new types of information, including genetic information. The Internet is growing rapidly, some would say chaotically. Locating the information you need can be like looking for that proverbial needle buried somewhere in a huge and ever-expanding haystack. Some good starting points are given in the Appendix (Section IV).

At several Internet "sites" or "addresses," consumers can acquire a basic foundation of information about genetic disorders from the educational material put out by government agencies, research groups, and lay organizations. By regularly checking these sites, they can keep current with new findings. As with any reference source, it is wise to take note of the credentials of those offering the information and how recent the information is.

Some sites are set up to enable consumers to communicate with each other on subjects of mutual interest. These are called *discussion groups* or *news groups.* Messages sent out by a person writing at one computer appear on the computer screens of all the people who have signed up to be in the group. Any reactions and comments are distributed electronically to all the group members. Consumers with a common interest in a genetic disorder can use the discussion group as a forum for asking questions of their own and for offering suggestions to others. Because a group brings many people together, it makes it possible for information obtained by one member to be readily shared with others. Although it is not their only purpose, these groups can be the means of keeping consumers informed about new genetic tests as they appear and about new types of treatments as they become available.

Person-to-Person Encounters

For some consumers, family and friends are a sufficient support system. For many others, however, contact with people facing similar situations is necessary for overcoming their feelings of isolation. Such contact may also enable them to get information they need to help them deal with any difficult practical problems. With people who are in the same boat, it is possible to speak openly, to obtain psychological support, and to share ideas easily. Consumers are spared having to make the explanations that are so often required when talking with outsiders.

Support groups are important mechanisms for establishing such contact. Members of a support group meet on a regular basis, and sometimes are assisted by a professionally trained facilitator. Support groups can be started in many ways. Frequently, hospitals and voluntary health organizations make all the arrangements. Newsletters of such organizations publish announcements that a group has been formed and invite new members to join. Many people have also started support groups on their own. Several organizations provide valuable assistance in locating or forming support groups (see Section III of the Appendix). Almost all support groups occasionally plan programs to examine new research findings. The support group members can then share this information with the genetic grapevines of which they are a part.

Helpful as they are, support groups are not suited to everyone. Support groups, either for single-gene disorders or complex disorders, seem to work best when all the individuals with the disorder are in the same stage of an illness. It can happen that the needs and concerns of the majority of the group do not coincide with one's own. Sometimes the meetings are inconvenient to get to because of distance or because of the time selected. There may be no time for meetings if one's daily schedule is filled and subject to unexpected changes. Or the need for such a group may vary, more necessary at some times than at others.

An alternative means of establishing contact is by *networking* to find just one or a few other individuals or families. Once the connection is made, it may be possible to set up ways to meet informally that will be mutually convenient if the distance is small, or to stay in touch via mail and by phone if it is not. Of course, the main difficulty is finding others whose situation is similar. This is especially the case when the disorder is a rare one.

Several of the organizations that work with consumers to find and set up support groups also help in setting up person-to-person matches. MUMS (Mothers United for Moral Support, Inc.), with its large database and its contacts with other voluntary health organizations, regularly assists in such efforts. Notices placed by consumers in the MUMS newsletter and in magazines (such as *Exceptional Parent*) were cited by consumers as effective in enabling them to locate others. One woman remains in close communication with a friend made through a notice she placed in the MUMS newsletter. They live at opposite ends of the country and have never met. However, they talk and write often. This friend gives her comfort and good advice. She believes that her friend receives similar benefits from her.

Computers are also opening up a new means of staying in touch by making it possible to communicate by *electronic mail*. Electronic mail (or e-mail) allows a note written by someone in one location to be received, almost instantly, by someone at another. The note will be seen whenever the person for whom it is intended turns on his or her computer and checks for e-mail. E-mail is quicker than regular mail and cheaper than long-distance telephone. It enables consumers to stay in close touch no matter what their time zone or how complicated their daily schedules. Whatever form the communication takes, the joining together of people from two different genetic grapevines can be the means of transferring useful information from one to the other.

Growth of the Genetic Grapevine

As more genes are found, their functions understood, and their association with illness recognized, a wide array of opportunities for genetic testing will arise. As this happens, the family genetic grapevine is likely to expand its presence as a means of education, communication, and assistance in making decisions about the use of such tests. The genetic grapevine is not a substitute for the traditional pathway of medical communication or for the activities of professionals directly involved in providing genetic services. It is, however, an invaluable—and inevitable—alternative pathway for information and assistance. Both the medical and the family pathways are important. And in the years to come, both must be strengthened.

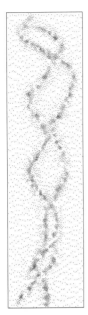

Chapter Nine

Some Thoughts and Recommendations

I t does not take a crystal ball to see that, in the years to come, many more genetic tests will become available. With the momentum generated by the Human Genome Project, tests of all kinds—for single-gene disorders as well as for complex multifactorial disorders—will be added to an already lengthening list. The scope of testing could even expand to include genes that may have a bearing on personality traits, behavioral patterns, or sexual preference.

Serious inadequacies and disturbing problems have arisen even at our current—and still relatively modest—level of genetic testing. These difficulties are certain to intensify as the number of genetic tests grows. The combined experiences and insights of consumers and genetic professionals reveal three areas that need prompt attention if we are to be prepared for the surge of genetic tests headed our way.

Recommendation 1: Consumers need accurate genetic information at the very beginning of their awareness of a genetic problem.

Though the starting point varies, it is usually from a physician that people first learn that they or a family member have a genetic disorder.

Thus it is that member of the medical community—whether a family doctor, a doctor at a walk-in clinic, or a specialist—who bears the primary responsibility for recognizing when genetic issues are involved and for providing the initial explanation about the genetic basis of the illness. Physicians are also responsible for referring their patients to the appropriate genetic professionals or genetic counseling groups where more detailed information can be provided and where testing (if so chosen) can be arranged. No one should be abandoned and left to search for needed explanations all alone. Up to now, this has occurred all too often. No clamor for "cost containment" or pressure to push through more patients per day can excuse a health-care provider from the obligation to deliver crucial information. That information is essential for informing the patient's options and actions. It is a basic and critical component of the doctor/patient relationship.

Fears have been raised that genetic testing is rampant and is being foisted on people whether they want it or not. When it comes to the newest form of genetic testing, DNA testing, the situation is quite different. Many doctors appear to be unaware of what the genetic basis of illness is and of what genetic tests are available. Even tests which have been in place for a long time, such as those for the sickle-cell, thalassemia, and Tay-Sachs genes, are not being discussed with consumers who are at risk for these disorders. The Human Genome Project, rather than inundating consumers with innumerable genetic tests, may just add to the number of genetic tests that physicians neither know about nor feel comfortable discussing.

The problems that consumers have had in getting genetic information at an early stage have often been blamed on the fact that medical schools have consistently shortchanged their students in the area of genetics. This can no longer be tolerated. Medical education will need to get serious about genetics and equip young doctors (of *all* stripes) with knowledge of basic genetic concepts and of the practical application of genetics in health care. Older physicians whose education did not include genetics need to get some training. The education of other health-care professionals, particularly nurses and nurse-midwives, must also include a firm grounding in genetics. Their work on the front lines in hospital and public-health settings puts them in a vitally important position to identify genetic matters and to direct patients to appropriate sources of information.

Not only the information itself, but also the manner in which it is given, is important. Medical education needs to stress better ways of giving bad news. Consumers have reported that they were first told of genetic problems far too bluntly, without any sensitivity to their feelings. Stories of doctors making a diagnosis and then turning on their heels and walking out of the room are not uncommon. It is never easy to be the messenger of disturbing news. But helping patients negotiate the emotional ordeal is not only humane, it is a necessary part of the process of enabling patients to think more clearly and to take in the information that they and their family members need.

The medical community has heard these calls before. What it perhaps has failed to recognize is that the absence of accurate genetic information not only jeopardizes the individual patient but also all the others in the family who are destined to learn from that patient. The harm done from lack of information can be extensive. Given the already daunting demands of medical education, the medical community has its work cut out.

Recommendation 2: Consumers need to have access to genetic services and to more kinds of educational tools as they make decisions about genetic tests.

In the years to come, more individuals whose family history indicates the possible presence of a faulty gene will be offered DNA tests. Even in the absence of a family history, tests for genes that can predispose to illnesses may become part of a standard package of medical tests. Commercial laboratories are already actively marketing DNA tests and are hard at work on developing approaches that will allow tests for a large number of different genetic predispositions to be carried out on one blood sample. However, no desire for quick answers and no eagerness for big profits justifies regarding genetic tests as simply another routine medical procedure.

Genetic testing raises many thorny issues and has profound

implications for consumers and for their family members. It should not be entered into without careful explanation. It should not be entered into without sufficient time allowed for someone to decide whether or not this is a test that should be done. This means that more professionals will be needed to deliver genetic services and better methods will be needed to communicate genetic information to consumers.

The present number of genetic specialists and genetic counselors will not be sufficient to meet the expected demand for genetic services. Currently there are about twenty programs that train master's level genetic counselors. More such programs should be created. Additional sources of qualified people should come from programs that prepare nurses, social workers, psychologists, and others to function as part of the genetic counseling team. Efforts to establish programs to train "single-gene counselors" (who can work in specialized areas such as sickle-cell anemia or breast cancer testing) should be encouraged. Genetic services groups in the U.S. and Canada that have initiated innovative training programs on a pilot basis have reported success both in enlarging the pool of genetics educators, especially in rural areas, and in remaining as a resource for them. Clearly more attention must be given to exploring all of these new modes of professional education and interaction. Careful evaluation of their strengths and weaknesses must occur now if the necessary professional infrastructure is to be in place in time to meet future needs.

What must also be set up is the regulatory infrastructure to make sure that DNA tests are valid and that they are performed properly. The task of setting up a regulatory framework is complicated. The Health Care Financing Administration has the authority to establish standards for laboratories that provide genetic tests. The Food and Drug Administration has the authority to evaluate and approve the tests themselves. Now is the time for the federal government to act, through these agencies, so that health-care providers and consumers can have confidence in the tests.

Whatever their training, professionals engaged in providing genetic services will need to make their communication with consumers more effective and informative. Consumers have repeatedly emphasized that verbal explanations alone are woefully inadequate, sometimes useless. Written materials are essential for summarizing information and enhancing understanding. Consumers are calling for printed materials, pertinent to their individual case, that they can take home and study. They would also welcome the opportunity to borrow items such as videotapes or CD-ROMs that they can watch at their leisure and that they can share with other family members. All of these materials are vital aids in enabling consumers to understand their situation and in helping them come to their own decisions about genetic testing.

Though members of the clergy often play a significant role in life-cycle events (birth, marriage, and death), they currently play a very limited role in dealing with genetic issues or assisting with any type of genetic decision. If they wish to be of help to parishioners facing such problems, religious institutions should consider including genetics in their programs for educating and preparing the future ministry.

Recommendation 3: Better methods of keeping consumers informed over time are essential.

Genetics research is a dynamic field. Knowledge about genes, and about ways of testing for genes connected with genetic illness, is continually expanding. Unless consumers keep abreast of these changes, they could be basing decisions for themselves and their children on outdated information. The relatives who depend on the family genetic grapevine could be relying on information that is incomplete. Too often, genetic information received at some point in the past becomes the bedrock of all future decisions and actions. Substantial efforts on many fronts need to be devoted to creating mechanisms that enable people to have access to the best available information on the genetic matters important to them.

A number of approaches, such as the ones indicated below, should be instituted so that consumers can be reached in several different ways:

- *The medical genetics community needs to develop methods to recontact patients in order to give them new findings about the genes for their disorder and any genetic test options that may have become available.*

Whether physicians are ever obligated to recontact former patients and provide them with newly gained information related to their health is a topic of debate. For most medical matters this is not a major issue. A person with a health problem should be able to learn the latest information and obtain the most current treatments in any doctor's office. Dr. Jones in Oregon does not have to spend time locating Mary Smith, a former patient of his who has moved to Virginia, to tell her about a newly approved medication that can treat her high blood pressure. Both Dr. Jones and Ms. Smith can expect that whichever physician she now goes to will tell her.

However, while someone with a health problem (such as high blood pressure) is usually under the care of a physician, someone needing genetic information may have no immediate health problem and not be under the care of a physician. And those who have had genetic counseling usually do not maintain a continuing relationship with the counseling team in the way they do with their family doctor. Therefore genetic information needs to be available separately from immediate treatment needs or crisis situations. The medical community must find ways to convey this information, as it evolves, to consumers.

One way to accomplish this is through the use of computer-based information storage and retrieval systems. Such systems could be set up in doctors' offices, hospitals, or specialty clinics. Once set up, they could be used to identify different groups of patients who wish to be kept informed about relevant genetic advances and about any new types of tests or treatments as they become available. Researchers could use computer systems to reach those individuals who have been part of their own studies. So could those who coordinate registries. Of course, it is unreasonable to expect any medical practitioner or genetic professional to spend the countless hours necessary to track down former patients who have moved, married, or remarried. For any system of continuous updating to succeed, consumers need to take the responsibility for supplying their current addresses and phone numbers so that they can be readily reached. Procedures for ensuring the privacy of all the individuals on the distribution list would be absolutely necessary.

- *Lay-led voluntary health organizations should intensify their educational efforts.*

Organizations positioned to reach a large number of individuals and families with a particular genetic interest should increase their role in the dissemination of genetic information. Newsletters, informational mailings, videotapes, and news made available via the Internet are all effective ways of communicating. Not all of the materials prepared should be limited to basic, introductory information. There need to be materials written for consumers who want more detailed information on genetic aspects, or who have special interests such as finding governmental or community programs they can tap into for assistance and services.

In addition, more emphasis should be given to arranging educational meetings and seminars for the lay person. Many consumers welcome the opportunity to meet with scientists and medical specialists and to hear explanations given in nontechnical language. Consumers have strongly recommended that, when such meetings are planned, groups be small in size and the information provided be tightly focused on the needs of a specific group. Consumers do not want to spend time traveling to a meeting that deals with topics not directly related to their situation.

- *Support groups and other organizations could further assist in making person-to-person contact possible and in enabling people to collect and consider genetic information.*

Through the impressive efforts of support groups, people facing similar circumstances have been put in touch with each other. Such efforts are extremely important. At present, however, some consumers cannot take advantage of these contacts because of the expense involved. Support groups and philanthropic organizations should work together to establish programs that subsidize travel costs, long-distance telephone charges, or charges for computer access to the Internet and electronic mail.

Religious and other institutions could also take the lead in helping to establish programs of respite care. Respite care programs enable parents and family members who look after individuals affected with an illness to have some time off. Most medical and social services focus on the person with a disorder but ignore the toll exacted on those who have taken on substantial caregiving obligations. Health insurance policies do not pay for this type of service. Among the many benefits of respite care is that it provides people with valuable time to gather information and to calmly consider their options.

As we can see, there is much to do before genetic testing becomes more widely available. The tasks ahead of us are of great importance. Time is short. We dare not delay.

A Final Word

In the garden of the Royal Summer Palace in Prague is the sculpture *Victory.* Victory is represented as a buoyant young man. His arms are raised upward—exultant, triumphant. But his exuberant figure is poised precariously on the edge of a precipice. So it is with any victory. The good fortune of one moment may set the stage for the misfortune of the next. The fruits of success contain the seeds of future problems and sometimes even disasters. Scientific research is now giving us powerful insights into our genes, making it possible to reveal our previously unknown and unimagined genetic secrets. If we are to derive real and enduring benefit from these scientific victories, we must be alert to the problems that this knowledge may create. And we must be prepared to confront these problems with caring, creativity, and courage.

Appendix
Resources for Consumers

The information listed in this Appendix can change over time. A link to an updated list of these resources can be found on the Internet at: http://www.cis.vt.edu/pages/zallen

I. Ways to Reach Centers Providing Genetic Services

Council of Regional Networks for Genetic Services (CORN)
Emory University, Pediatrics/Medical Genetics
2040 Ridgewood Drive
Atlanta, Georgia 30322
Telephone: 404-727-1475
FAX: 404-727-1827
Internet address: http://www.cc.emory.edu/PEDIATRICS/corn/corn.htm

National Society of Genetic Counselors
233 Canterbury Drive
Wallingford, Pennsylvania 19806-6617

II. Ways to Reach Voluntary Health Organizations

The groups listed in this section can direct consumers to organizations where information about a particular disorder can be obtained. In addition, the groups listed often provide their own printed materials and use their own databases to conduct searches for information about disorders, tests, and current treatments. Some of them assist in putting consumers in contact with support groups, or networks, or with centers providing genetic services. (See Section III below for other ways to find support groups.) Internet addresses, where available, are also shown. The first two organizations listed cover the broadest range of genetic disorders.

United States

Alliance of Genetic Support Groups
   35 Wisconsin Circle, Suite 440
   Chevy Chase, Maryland 20815
   Telephone: 800-336-4363 or 301-652-5553
   FAX: 301-654-0171
   Internet address: http://medhelp.org/www/agsg.htm

National Organization for Rare Disorders (NORD)
   P.O. Box 8923
   New Fairfield, Connecticut 06812
   Telephone: 800-999-6673 or 203-746-6518
   FAX: 203-746-6481
   TTD: 203-746-6927
   Internet address: http://www.nord-rdb.com/~orphan

March of Dimes Birth Defects Foundation
   1275 Mamaroneck Avenue
   White Plains, NY 10605
   Telephone: 888-663-4637; 914-428-7100
   FAX: 914-428-8203
   Internet address: http://www.modimes.org

*National Center for Education in Maternal and Child Health
(NCEMCH)*
   2000 15th Street North, Suite 701
   Arlington, Virginia 22201
   Telephone: 703-524-7802
   FAX: 703-524-9335

National Health Information Center (NHIC)
   Department of Health and Human Services
   P.O. Box 1133
   Washington, D.C. 20013
   Telephone: 800-336-4797; 301-565-4167
   FAX: 301-984-4256
   Internet address: http://nhic-nt.health.org

*National Information Center for Children and Youth with
Disabilities (NICHCY)*
   P.O. Box 1492
   Washington, D.C. 20013
   Telephone: 800-695-0285; 202-884-8200 (TDD and voice for both)
   FAX: 202-884-8441
   Internet address: http://www.aed.org/nichcy

Boys Town National Research Hospital (for Hereditary Deafness)
   555 N. 30th Street
   Omaha, Nebraska 68131
   Telephone: 800-835-1468 (TDD and voice); 402-498-6622

American Cancer Society
   Telephone: 800-ACS-2345
   Internet address: http://www.cancer.org

National Cancer Institute (National Institutes of Health), Cancer Information Center
   Telephone: 800-422-6237
   Internet address: http://cancernet.nci.nih.gov

National Alliance of Breast Cancer Organizations
   9 East 37th Street, 10th floor
   New York, New York 10016
   Telephone: 800-719-9154

Y-ME National Breast Cancer Organization
   212 W. Van Buren Street
   Chicago, Illinois 60607
   Telephone: 800-221-2141; 312-986-8338; 312-986-9505 (Spanish)
   Internet address: http://www.y-me.org

Canada

Canadian Directory of Genetic Support Groups
   Provincial IODE Genetics Resource Centre
   800 Commissioners Road East
   London, Ontario N6C 2V5 Canada
   Telephone: 519-685-8453; 800-243-8416 (Ontario only)
   Internet address:
      http://www.lhsc.on.ca/programs/medgenet/support.htm

United Kingdom

Genetic Interest Group (GIG)
   Farringdon Point, 29-35 Farringdon Road
   London, England EC1M 3JB
   Telephone: (0171) 430-0090
   FAX: (0171) 430-0092
   Electronic mail: 101366.760@compuserve.com

Research Trust for Metabolic Diseases in Children (RTMDC)
   Golden Gates Lodge, Weston Road, Crewe
   Cheshire, England CW1 1XN
   Telephone: (01270) 250221
   FAX: (01270) 250244

III. Ways to Reach Peer Support Groups

The organizations listed in this section help consumers contact support groups. If no group exists at a convenient travel distance, the organizations frequently provide assistance to consumers interested in organizing such groups. They may also help in making one-to-one matches.

United States

American Self-Help Clearinghouse
Northwest Covenant Medical Center
25 Pocono Road
Denville, New Jersey 07834
Telephone: 201-625-9565
FAX: 201-625-8848
TDD: 201-625-9053

MUMS, Mothers United for Moral Support, Inc., National Parent-to-Parent Network
150 Custer Court
Green Bay, Wisconsin 54301
Telephone: 414-336-5333
FAX: 414-339-0995

National Parent-to-Parent Support and Information System
P.O. Box 907
Blue Ridge, Georgia 30513
Telephone: 800-651-1151; 706-632-8822
FAX: 706-632-8830
Internet address: http://www.nppsis.org

National Self-Help Clearinghouse
25 West 43rd Street, Suite 620
New York, New York 10036
Telephone: 212-354-8525
FAX: 212-642-1956

Exceptional Parent
555 Kinderkamack Road
Oradell, New Jersey 07649-1517
Telephone: 800-372-7368
FAX: 201-634-6599
Internet address: http://www.familyeducation.com
    Click on "Special Needs," then on "Search & Respond."
This is a magazine with a "Search & Respond" column. Consumers can write in (by regular mail or Internet) and locate other readers interested in the same health issues. The magazine can be reached at its editorial offices.

Canada

Parent-to-Parent Link Programme
c/o Easter Seal Society
250 Ferrand Drive, Suite 200
Don Mills, Ontario, Canada M3C 3P2
Telephone: 416-421-8778, extension 334; 416-421-8377;
   800-668-6252 (Ontario only)

United Kingdom

Contact a Family
170 Tottenham Court Road
London, England W1P 0HA
Telephone: 0171 383-3555
FAX: 0171 383-0259
Electronic mail: specific_cond@cafamily.org.uk

IV. Ways to Find Genetic Information on the Internet

This section provides addresses on the Internet where a search for genetic
information can begin. Internet addresses appearing in Section II above are
also good starting points. It is possible to connect from many of these
starting points to other resources on the Internet. New resources appear
all the time, and addresses can change. Consumers may seek the most
current information by using various "search engines" such as Yahoo, Alta
Vista, Lycos, Excite, Infoseek, and Magellan.

GeneNet
Internet address: http://www.genenet.com
Primarily for professionals in the genetics community, this site connects
with other Internet resources of use to consumers.

Genetics Education Center Homepage
Internet address: http://www.kumc.edu/GEC/
This page contains a useful compilation of many different sources of
information related to human genetics and medical genetics.

Genline
Internet address: http://www.hslib.washington.edu/genline
This site is allied with Helix, a national directory of DNA diagnostic
laboratories, and provides information about genetic disorders and genetic
testing to clinicians. It contains material that will be of interest to consumers as well. It is still in development, so only a few genetic disorders
may be described.

The Human Molecular Genetics Network
    Internet address: http://www.informatik.uni-rostock.de/HUM-MOLGEN
    This location serves as a forum for information on molecular genetics
    and genetic disorders. Subscriptions are free. Special procedures are
    followed to protect consumer privacy when requests for information
    and referral are received. You don't have to be a subscriber to post a
    request.

Med Help International
    Internet address: http://www.medhelp.org
    This is a comprehensive site for patient education materials in lay language,
    access to libraries of medical information, and public forums on specific
    issues.

Medical Matrix. A Guide to Internet Clinical Medical Resources
    Internet address: http://www.slackinc.com/matrix/PATIENT.HTML

MedWeb Biomedical Internet Resources
    Internet address: http://www.gen.emory.edu/MEDWEB/

*National Institutes of Health, National Center for Human Genome
Research*
    Internet address: http://www.nchgr.nih.gov
    This page comes with links to scientific and technical information. Increas-
    ingly, more links to consumer and lay public materials are being included.

National Institutes of Health, National Cancer Institute
    Internet addresses:
        gopher://gopher.nih.gov:70/11/clin/cancernet/pdqinfo
        http://cancernet.nci.nih.gov
    This site is the access point for CancerNet, a database containing infor-
    mation on all types of cancer.

National Institutes of Health, Office of Rare Disease Research
    Internet address: http://rarediseases.info.nih.gov/ord/pages
    A rare disease clinical research database for inherited and acquired rare
    or orphan diseases and conditions

NOAH: New York Online Access to Health
    Internet address: http://www.noah.cuny.edu/
    Genetic information is included among the kinds of consumer health
    information that can be reached at this site. Material is presented in
    Spanish as well as English.

Online Mendelian Inheritance in Man (OMIM)
    Internet address: http://www3.ncbi.nlm.nih.gov/Omim
    This is the Internet version of a classic reference, *Mendelian Inheritance
    in Man* (edited by Victor McKusick). Every known genetic disorder is
    included. The material is not presented in lay terms and the references
    cited are generally available only in medical libraries.

V. *Other Resources for Consumers*

Equal Employment Opportunities Commission
Office of Communications and Legislative Affairs
1801 L Street, NW
Washington, D.C. 20507
Telephone: 800-669-4000; 800-669-EEOC (publications and referral);
    800-800-3302 (TDD)
This is the federal agency which oversees the employment provisions of
the Americans with Disabilities Act.

Council for Responsible Genetics
5 Upland Road, Suite 3
Cambridge, Massachusetts, 02140
Telephone: 617-868-0870
FAX: 617-491-5344
Internet address: http://www.essential.org/crg/
A main interest of this organization is in countering genetic discrimination.
The organization can provide information to consumers on the status
in their state of protective legislation against genetic discrimination in
insurance and employment.

National Association of Insurance Commissioners
Suite 1100, 120 West 12th Street
Kansas City, Missouri 64105
Telephone: 816-842-3600
This group can refer consumers to the insurance commission in their states
where information on insurance policy can be obtained.

*Multilingual Catalog of Patient Education Materials on Genetic and
Related Maternal/Child Health Topics*
This catalog was developed by the Center for Human and Molecular
Genetics of the New Jersey Medical School as a resource for health
professionals. Consumers can use it to find out where relevant materials,
published in a variety of languages, can be obtained. The catalog is available, free of charge, through the Maternal and Child Health Clearinghouse,
2070 Chain Bridge Road, Vienna, Virginia 22182. Telephone: 703-821-8955;
FAX: 703-821-2098.

National Library of Medicine, National Institutes of Health
The National Library of Medicine (NLM) is the U.S. national repository
of biomedical information and materials. The NLM has developed a number of computer-based reference tools. One of these tools, MEDLINE®,
can be used to search through a vast number of scientific and medical journals to find publications on specific topics. Another tool, a database
known as the Directory of Information Resources Online or DIRLINE®,
can be used to search out organizations, research projects, government

agencies, and other places that provide information on specific genetic disorders. PDQ® is the cancer information database.

Many public and medical libraries have the capacity to connect to the NLM and to access these NLM reference tools. Consumers with a computer can also access the NLM databases on their own. To do this, they must set up an account with the NLM. There is no charge for an account. There is also available special user-friendly software, called GRATEFUL MED®, which simplifies the search process. This software is available for purchase through the National Technical Information Service, U.S. Department of Commerce, 5285 Port Royal Road, Springfield, Virginia 22161; Telephone: 800-423-9255.

Consumers with GRATEFUL MED® software on their computer can reach the NLM databases in two ways. They can dial in with a modem. Or they can access these databases through the Internet if they also have Telnet software installed on their computer or available through their commercial computer network.

Consumers without GRATEFUL MED® software can reach NLM databases on the Internet if they have World Wide Web Browser Netscape 3.0 or higher. The Internet address is: http://www.nlm.nih.gov.

In any case, an account with NLM is necessary. DIRLINE searches are free. There is a charge for searching MEDLINE and other databases. The costs depend on the amount of information that is viewed, printed, and downloaded. Cost of the average search ranges from $1.25 to $5. There are no monthly or long-distance charges. Billing is done quarterly.

For further information, contact: MEDLARS Management Section, National Library of Medicine, 8600 Rockville Pike, Bethesda, Maryland 20894. Telephone: 800-638-8480.

Suggested Further Reading

On Genetics and Health Issues

Anderson, W. French. 1995. "Gene Therapy." *Scientific American* (September) pp. 124–128.

Cavenee, Webster K., and Raymond L. White. 1995. "The Genetic Basis of Cancer." *Scientific American* (March) pp. 72–79.

Gelehrter, Thomas D., and Francis S. Collins. 1990. *Principles of Medical Genetics.* Baltimore: Williams & Wilkins.

Gonick, Larry, and Mark Wheelis. 1991. *The Cartoon Guide to Genetics* (updated edition). New York: Harper Perennial, HarperCollins Publishers. (Available through HarperCollins Publishers, P.O. Box 588, Dunmore, Pa. 18512. 1-800-331-3761. ISBN: 0-06-273099-1)

Hodgson, S. V., and E. R. Maher. 1993. *A Practical Guide to Human Cancer Genetics.* New York: Cambridge University Press.

Mange, Elaine Johansen, and Arthur P. Mange. 1994. *Basic Human Genetics.* Sunderland, Mass.: Sinauer Associates, Inc.

Nelson-Anderson, Danette L., and Cynthia V. Waters. 1995. *Genetic Connections: A Guide to Documenting Your Individual and Family Health History.* Washington, Mo.: Sonters Publishing.

Pierce, Benjamin A. 1990. *The Family Genetic Sourcebook.* New York: John Wiley & Sons, Inc.

Selkoe, Dennis J. 1991. "Amyloid Protein and Alzheimer's Disease." *Scientific American* (November) pp. 68–78.

Wynbrandt, James, and Mark D. Ludman. 1991. *The Encyclopedia of Genetic Disorders and Birth Defects.* New York: Facts on File, Inc.

On Ethical, Legal, and Social Aspects of Genetic Testing

Ad Hoc Committee on Genetic Testing/Insurance Issues. 1995. "Background Statement: Genetic Testing and Insurance." *American Journal of Human Genetics* 56:327–331.

American Society of Human Genetics/American College of Medical Genetics Report. 1995. "Points to Consider: Ethical, Legal, and Psychological Implications of Genetic Testing in Children and Adolescents." *American Journal of Human Genetics* 57:1233–1241.

Andrews, Lori B., Jane E. Fullarton, Neil A. Holtzman, and Arno G. Motulsky, eds. (Committee on Assessing Genetic Risks, Division of Health Sciences Policy, Institute of Medicine). 1994. *Assessing Genetic Risks: Implications for Health and Social Policy.* Washington, D.C.: National Academy Press.

Annas, George J., and Sherman Elias, eds. 1992. *Gene Mapping: Using Law and Ethics as Guides.* New York: Oxford University Press.

Billings, Paul R., Mel A. Kohn, Margaret de Cuevas, Jonathan Beckwith, Joseph S. Alper, and Marvin R. Natowicz. 1992. "Discrimination as a Consequence of Genetic Testing." *American Journal of Human Genetics* 50:476–482.

Clarke, Angus, ed., *Genetic Counseling: Practice and Principles.* London and New York: Routledge.

Cordori, Ann-Marie, and Jason Brandt. 1994. "Psychological Costs and Benefits of Predictive Testing for Huntington's Disease." *American Journal of Medical Genetics* 54:174–184.

Cranor, Carl F., ed. 1994. *Are Genes Us?* New Brunswick, N.J.: Rutgers University Press.

Duster, Troy. 1990. *Backdoor to Eugenics.* London and New York: Routledge.

Hubbard, Ruth, and Elijah Wald. 1997. *Exploding the Gene Myth.* Boston: Beacon Press.

Huggins, Marlene, Maurice Bloch, Shelin Kanani, Oliver W. J. Quarrell, Jane Theilmann, Amy Hedrick, Bernard Dickens, Abbyann Lynch, and Michael Hayden. 1990. "Ethical and Legal Dilemmas Arising during Predictive Testing for Adult-Onset Disease: The Experience of Huntington Disease." *American Journal of Human Genetics* 47:4–12.

Kevles, Daniel J., and Leroy Hood, eds. 1992. *The Code of Codes: Scientific and Social Issues in the Human Genome Project.* Cambridge, Mass.: Harvard University Press.

Lippman, Abby. 1993. "Prenatal Genetic Testing and Geneticization: Mother Matters for All." *Fetal Diagnosis and Therapy* 8 (suppl 1):175–188.

Nelkin, Dorothy, and Laurence Tancredi. 1989. *Dangerous Diagnostics: The Social Power of Biological Information.* New York: Basic Books, Inc.

Nelson, J. Robert. 1994. *On the New Frontiers of Genetics and Religion.* Grand Rapids, Mich.: William B. Eerdmans Publishing Company.

Paul, Diane B. 1995. *Controlling Human Heredity: 1865 to the Present.* Atlantic Highlands, N.J.: Humanities Press.

Quaid, Kimberly A., and Michael Morris. 1993. "Reluctance to Undergo Predictive Testing: The Case of Huntington Disease." *American Journal of Medical Genetics* 45:41–45.

Reardon, W., J. F. Floyd, J. Myring, L. P. Lazarou, A. L. Meredith, and P. S. Harper. 1992. "Five Years Experience of Predictive Testing for Myotonic Dystrophy Using Linked DNA Markers." *American Journal of Medical Genetics* 43:1006–1011.

Rennie, John. 1994. "Grading the Gene Tests." *Scientific American* (June) pp. 88–97.

Weiss, Joan O., and Jayne S. Mackta. 1996. *Starting and Sustaining Genetic Support Groups.* Baltimore: Johns Hopkins University Press.

Wertz, Dorothy C., Joanna H. Fanos, and Philip R. Reilly. 1994. "Genetic Testing for Children and Adolescents: Who Decides?" *JAMA, Journal of the American Medical Association* 272:875–881.

Wertz, Dorothy C., and John C. Fletcher, eds. 1989. *Ethics and Human Genetics: A Cross-Cultural Perspective.* New York: Springer-Verlag.

Wiggins, Sandi, Patti Whyte, Marlene Huggins, Shelin Adam, Jane Theilmann, Maurice Bloch, Samuel B. Sheps, Martin T. Schechter, and Michael R. Hayden. 1992. "The Psychological Consequences of Predictive Testing for Huntington's Disease." *The New England Journal of Medicine* 327:1401–1405.

Working Party of the Clinical Genetics Society (UK) Report. 1994. "The Genetic Testing of Children." *Journal of Medical Genetics* 31:785–797.

Glossary

amniocentesis A procedure, usually carried out at about the sixteenth week of pregnancy, that obtains a sample of the fluid (amniotic fluid) surrounding the fetus. The fluid is collected by insertion of a needle through the mother's abdominal wall and into the sac immediately surrounding the fetus. Studies of the fluid and the fetal cells contained within it can provide information about the fetus's chromosomes, genes, and chemical makeup.

autosomal dominant A pattern of inheritance attributed to genes located on chromosomes other than the X and Y (sex) chromosomes. The trait or disorder will appear even when only one copy of the gene for that trait or disorder is present. Males and females are equally likely to be affected, and the trait can show up in successive generations of a family.

autosomal recessive A pattern of inheritance attributed to genes located on chromosomes other than the X and Y (sex) chromosomes. Both copies of the gene in a gene pair must be flawed for a disorder to appear. Males and females are equally likely to be affected. The disorder can appear suddenly with no prior history of it in the family.

autosome Any chromosome that is not part of the pair of sex chromosomes. Humans have twenty-two pairs of autosomes, numbered from 1 to 22.

base Any one of the four units—adenine (A), guanine (G), thymine (T), and cytosine (C)—found in a DNA molecule. The order (sequence) of the bases along one strand of the DNA molecule provides information for assembling proteins. The bases on one DNA strand pair up with the bases on the other DNA strand (A with T, G with C), providing stability to the DNA molecule.

carrier An individual who has a gene pair in which one of the genes is flawed. The presence of the flawed gene is masked by the dominant functional gene.

carrier test A genetic test performed to determine if a healthy individual has a flawed gene which, if expressed in his or her children, could lead to a genetic disorder.

cell The basic building block of all organisms. The human body is composed of trillions of cells, specialized into many cell types including muscle, nerve, blood, bone, and skin cells.

chorionic villus sampling A procedure, usually carried out between the ninth and twelfth weeks of pregnancy, to collect cells from placental tissue. Samples can be taken in several ways. Studies of these cells can yield information about fetal chromosomes and genes.

chromosome A long ribbon-like structure containing collections of genes. Each chromosome is a long thread of DNA. The standard number of chromosomes in humans is forty-six.

collagen One of the most abundant proteins produced in the human body. It is found in bone, cartilage, skin, and other places which provide structural support.

complex disorder A disorder attributed to a combination of genetic and environmental factors. Cancer, heart disease, diabetes, and many other common health problems fall into this category. (See also "multifactorial disorder.")

direct test A test that can detect specific mutations or alterations in the DNA of a gene.

DNA The abbreviation for deoxyribonucleic acid, the thread-like molecule that is the genetic material. DNA has the form of a double-stranded helix. Each strand contains a long sequence of four types of chemical bases (denoted as A, C, G, and T). The sequence of bases makes up the genetic code containing the information for all of the proteins that an organism can produce. The helix is held together by strand-to-strand bonds, following the chemical rule that A connects to T, and G connects to C. DNA is located in the chromosomes within the organism's cells.

dominant mutation A mutation whose effect is revealed even when it is present in only one of the genes in the gene pair.

enzyme protein A type of protein whose function is to act as a catalyst and make chemical reactions possible in living organisms. In the absence of the enzyme, the chemical reaction for which the enzyme is responsible will not take place.

exclusion test A form of genetic test in which fetal cells are examined to see whether they contain the same genetic markers that are present in a grandparent affected with a genetic disorder. This is done when the at-risk parent does not wish to know his or her own genetic status. If the fetus has inherited a marker from the affected grandparent, the fetus will have the same 50 percent risk of developing a dominant disorder as the at-risk parent. If the marker inherited is derived from the unaffected grandparent, the risk of developing the disorder is much lower.

gamete A male or female reproductive cell. In the female, an ovum (or egg); in the male, a sperm.

gene A defined section of DNA along the chromosome that encodes information for the production of a particular protein necessary for the functioning of the organism.

gene pair The two genes, one derived from each parent, with information for producing a protein. One gene comes from the chromosome set contributed by the egg cell; the other gene from the chromosome set contributed by the sperm cell. All genes come in pairs with the exception of genes on the X chromosome in males. Males have only one X chromosome; therefore the genes on the X chromosome in males are present only in a single dose.

gene therapy A means of treating or correcting genetic disorders by introducing the normal or functioning gene into the cells of individuals who lack the normal gene.

genetic counseling A multifaceted interaction between a genetic professional and a client in which information about individual and family genetic risks is provided along with related information about tests, treatments, and reproductive options.

genome The total genetic material contained in a full set of chromosomes of an organism.

hemoglobin The molecule that transports oxygen throughout the body. It is made up of four chains, two of one type of protein and two of another. Changes in either of the proteins can lead to impaired function, such as occurs in sickle-cell anemia.

"junk" DNA Stretches of DNA along the chromosomes that seem to have no known function.

karyotype An organized picture showing all of the chromosomes in a cell.

late-onset disorder A disorder which is not apparent at birth but develops later in the course of an individual's life.

linkage test An indirect form of genetic testing in which a known region of DNA located near a gene for a disorder can be used as a "marker"—or indicator—for that gene. This type of testing is used when the target gene has not yet been identified or when a direct test is not practical because the specific mutation is not known.

locus The position that a gene occupies on a chromosome.

marker A region of the chromosome that can be identified and followed as it is inherited. This can be a nearby gene which produces a known protein, a restriction enzyme break point, or a series of repeated bases.

multifactorial disorder A disorder which is brought on by the joint action of multiple factors. The contributing factors include several different genes as well as various types of agents from the environment. (See also "complex disorder.")

multiplex genetic test A genetic test in which a single blood (or tissue) sample is examined for many different types of mutations.

mutation Any permanent change or alteration in the genetic material (for example, in the DNA base sequence of a gene) that changes the nature of the product made under the direction of that gene.

noninformative result A situation in linkage testing in which no conclusions can be drawn. This can occur because there is insufficient information to determine which marker is associated with the genes of interest or because the same marker is associated with normal and mutant genes.

nucleus The place within the cell where the chromosomes are contained. It is separated from the rest of the cell by a porous membrane.

polymerase chain reaction (PCR) A laboratory technique that permits a small DNA section located between two fixed points on the DNA molecule to be duplicated many times, yielding many copies of that DNA section.

prenatal test A genetic test performed during pregnancy to obtain information about the chromosomes or genes of a fetus.

presymptomatic test A genetic test performed to determine if a gene (or genes) are present which will bring on a health problem later in an individual's life.

private mutation A mutation unique to a particular family.

probability The odds or chance that an event will happen.

protein A molecule composed of amino acids connected together in a linear fashion. The order (sequence) of the amino acids in a protein is determined by the order of bases found within the DNA of a gene.

recessive mutation A mutation whose effect is revealed only when it occurs in both genes of a gene pair.

regulatory protein Proteins that help control the activities of genes or that integrate the different chemical processes which occur in an organism.

repeats or repeated sequences A series of two or more DNA bases which occurs over and over in tandem at one place on a chromosome. Some disorders (such as Huntington disease, fragile-X syndrome, and myotonic muscular dystrophy) result when a three-base sequence (CAG in Huntington disease) recurs many times within a gene. In some cases, there can be an expansion in number of repeats in successive generations.

restriction enzyme A protein that breaks the chromosomes apart into many small fragments by cutting the DNA of the chromosomes wherever a specific short sequence of bases occurs.

sequence The linear order of the bases in the DNA molecule or of amino acids in a protein molecule.

sex chromosomes The X and Y chromosomes. Females have two X chromosomes; males have one X and one Y.

single-gene disorder A disorder which comes about when there is a mutation in a specific gene, and one (for a dominant disorder) or both (for a recessive disorder) of the genes in the gene pair cannot function properly.

somatic mutation A mutation which occurs in any of the body cells of an individual over the course of that person's life. Since the mutation is not in the eggs or the sperm cells, it cannot be passed on to children.

structural protein A type of protein whose function is to provide shape and support to the various parts of the organism.

susceptibility test A genetic test for a gene whose presence can increase the chances of developing a health problem later in life. The problem may no develop even if the damaged gene is present, and it may occur even if th gene is absent.

target gene A gene, associated with a disorder, that is being tracked wi the aid of markers closely linked to it.

tumor-suppressor gene One of a group of genes which functions in regulation of cell division. If both copies of the same gene are faulty, t an important step in the regulation may be missing, thus contributin the development of tumors.

X-linked dominant A pattern of inheritance attributed to genes locate the X chromosome. A disorder will appear when one copy of the ger that disorder is present. Affected males pass X-linked dominant ger all of their daughters but none of their sons. Affected females pass X- dominant genes, on average, to half of their daughters and half o sons.

X-linked recessive A pattern of inheritance attributed to genes loca the X chromosome. Males with the gene will be affected because genes on their single X chromosome will be expressed. Females, w two X chromosomes, can be carriers. Affected males in a fai related through females.

Index

Page numbers in boldface refer to glossary entries.

About the Author

Doris Teichler Zallen is Professor of Science-and-Technology Studies and Director of *Choices and Challenges,* a public humanities educational project, in the Center for Interdisciplinary Studies at Virginia Tech. She was educated at Brooklyn College and received her graduate degrees from Harvard University. A former laboratory scientist who has made contributions to cell biology and genetic linkage testing, she has turned her attention to the dynamic relationship that exists between scientific work and the cultural context from which the work emerges. Her recent research deals with the history of genetics and with science policy. She is co-editor of *Science and Morality: New Directions in Bioethics.* Zallen has been a member of the Recombinant DNA Advisory Committee (the RAC) of the National Institutes of Health and of its Human Gene Therapy Subcommittee. During her tenure on the RAC, she chaired the Working Group on Informed Consent.